Paul J. Rogers, M.D.
Columbus O.H.

RHYTHM QUIZLETS
SELF ASSESSMENT

SECOND EDITION

OHIO STATE UNIVERSITY MEDICAL BOOKSTORE
MARRIOTT
RHYTHM QUIZLETS SELF ASSESSMENT
DEPT:130 NR 0896
CAR
$32.95
9 780683 055825

OSU Bookstore
32.95 12/96

RHYTHM QUIZLETS
SELF ASSESSMENT

SECOND EDITION

HENRY J. L. MARRIOTT, M.D.

Director of Clinical Research and Education
Rogers Heart Foundation, Inc.
St. Petersburg, Florida
Clinical Professor of Medicine (Cardiology)
Emory University
Atlanta, Georgia

Clinical Professor of Pediatrics (Cardiology)
University of Florida, Gainesville, Florida

Clinical Professor of Medicine (Cardiology)
University of South Florida, Tampa, Florida

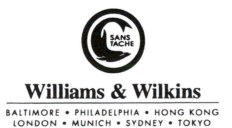

Williams & Wilkins

BALTIMORE • PHILADELPHIA • HONG KONG
LONDON • MUNICH • SYDNEY • TOKYO

A WAVERLY COMPANY

Editor: Jonathan W. Pine, Jr.
Managing Editor: Molly Mullen
Production Coordinator: Kimberly S. Nawrozki
Copy Editor: Pamela Goehrig
Designer: Norman W. Och
Illustration Planner: Lorraine Wrzosek
Typesetter: Automated Graphics
Printer: McNaughton & Gunn
Binder: McNaughton & Gunn

Copyright © 1996 Williams & Wilkins

351 West Camden Street
Baltimore, Maryland 21201-2436 USA

Rose Tree Corporate Center
1400 North Providence Road
Building II, Suite 5025
Media, Pennsylvania 19063-2043 USA

All rights reserved. This book is protected by copyright. No part of this book may be reproduced in any form or by any means, including photocopying, or utilized by any information storage and retrieval system without written permission from the copyright owner.

Accurate indications, adverse reactions and dosage schedules for drugs are provided in this book, but it is possible that they may change. The reader is urged to review the package information data of the manufacturers of the medications mentioned.

Printed in the United States of America

First Edition, 1987

Library of Congress Cataloging-in-Publication Data

Marriott, Henry J. L. (Henry Joseph Llewelyn), 1917–
    Rhythm quizlets: self assessment / Henry J. L. Marriott.—2nd ed.
       p.   cm.
    Includes bibliographical references and index.
    ISBN 0-683-05582-8
    1.   Arrhythmia—Diagnosis—Problems, exercises, etc.
    2.   Electrocardiography—Problems, exercises, etc. I. Title.
    RC685.A65M373 1996
    616.1'2807547'076—dc20   95-22628
                                                          CIP

The publishers have made every effort to trace the copyright holders for borrowed material. If they have inadvertently overlooked any, they will be pleased to make the necessary arrangements at the first opportunity.

95 96 97 98 99
1 2 3 4 5 6 7 8 9 10

Reprints of chapters may be purchased from Williams & Wilkins in quantities of 100 or more. Call Isabella Wise, Special Sales Department, (800) 358-3583.

RECYCLED

PREFACE TO THE SECOND EDITION

Since the previous edition, the routine recording of three simultaneous ECG leads has become the norm—a trend much to be welcomed and encouraged because it offers many potential benefits:

1. It is often diagnostically useful to observe the shape of certain beats in more than one lead at the same time (e.g., see Figures 42, 46, 157, and 161).
2. At times, a diagnosis can be made *only* if the same beat can be observed in two or more leads (see Figures 177, 234, 272, and 280).

3. There are three times as many chances of recognizing inconspicuous items, such as diminutive P waves or pacemaker spikes (see Figures 161 and 228).
4. If one lead is disturbed by artifact, there are two additional chances of obtaining an undisturbed baseline (see Figures 41 and 234).

The total number of arrhythmic tracings has been increased from 211 to 286, and of the new inclusions, more than half are presented with three or more simultaneous leads.

All of the ground rules laid out in the Preface to the First Edition apply to this updated and expanded version.

PREFACE TO THE FIRST EDITION

This volume is intended for those interested in learning how to recognize arrhythmias in the electrocardiogram or in sharpening their diagnostic skills. Without slavishly adhering to an order of increasing complexity, I have arranged the tracings in an approximate sequence of graduated sophistication. Everything from the simple extrasystole and the uncomplicated Wenckebach period to the concealed junctional extrasystole and concealed supernormal conduction is included, so that a perusal of each tracing from first to last provides a graded approach to virtually all of the arrhythmias.

I have divided the book into "zones." In the Green Zone, each tracing contains one or more straightforward disturbances of rhythm or conduction or both, all suitable for a beginner to learn from. On entering the Yellow Zone, however, one must tread warily: all the entries in this zone contain at least one pothole or detour that complicates the diagnostic quest. In the Red Zone, the territory is full of pitfalls and booby traps, consisting of advanced and intricate tracings, many of which require considerable knowledge and ingenuity to traverse.

All tracings are printed on the left page, whereas the interpretations are on the right, so they can be kept out of sight while studying the arrhythmia. "Diagnoses" are confined to the arrhythmias and blocks, and the main diagnostic features that should be considered in each example are stressed by boldface type. When an additional, nonarrhythmic diagnosis, such as chamber hypertrophy or myocardial infarction, is obvious, it has been added in parentheses. Nonspecific ST-T abnormalities are ignored.

In addition to the basic interpretation, often a special point or two exists to which attention should be drawn—a rationale for the diagnosis, a note about the mechanism of the arrhythmia, or a warning about a hidden trap. Comments addressed to such matters are included under a second heading, "Special Points."

Although the thrust of this text is diagnosis, whenever there is a threat of misguided therapy or if there seems to be some other good reason to do so, I have included a pertinent note on treatment.

In many of the simpler and in some of the more complex tracings, no special point is needed nor any compelling reason to comment on therapy. In these cases, only the bare bones of diagnosis are presented.

A few key references, ancient and modern, with which arrhythmophiles should be acquainted, are included.

Finally, it is my hope that the reader will find these rhythmic riddles both beguiling and instructive.

St. Petersburg, Florida   Henry J. L. Marriott

CONTENTS

GREEN ZONE
PAGE / 1

YELLOW ZONE
PAGE / 37

RED ZONE
PAGE / 157

ABBREVIATIONS AND LABELING

ABBREVIATIONS

The following abbreviations are widely used, and I have used them throughout the text without further explanation:

A-V = atrioventricular
I-V = intraventricular
BB = bundle branch
BBB = bundle-branch block
RBBB = right bundle-branch block
LBBB = left bundle-branch block
VPB = ventricular premature beat
APB = atrial premature beat
AIVR = accelerated idioventricular rhythm

INTERVALS

In dealing with clinical tracings at a paper speed of 25 mm/sec, I have avoided the modern affectation of using milliseconds—an affectation that introduces numerous unneeded zeros and is as meaningful as proffering Miss America's measurements in millimeters. Accordingly, intervals and cycle lengths in the text are recorded in decimal form (e.g., 0.36 sec) or as hundredths of a second (e.g., 36). All numbers inscribed on the tracings and in the laddergrams are hundredths of a second.

RATES

Rates, so often disregarded in clinical interpretations (how often have you heard the diagnosis "2:1 block" without any mention of rate) are of immense importance and have therefore been stressed in these interpretations. Conduction ratios are often overstressed at the expense of rate, although rates are far more important than ratios: for example, 2:1 block at an atrial rate of 72 is a disaster and has quite a different significance from 2:1 block at an atrial rate of 120, which may be a blessing.

LEAD LABELS

For simplicity's sake, the limb leads are generally labeled as follows:

Lead I	is labeled 1
II	2
III	3
aVR	R
aVL	L
aVF	F

Apart from the routine clinical leads, the following labels are used:

MCL_1 = modified CL_1, that is, positive electrode on chest at C_1 (V_1) position with negative electrode at left shoulder.

MCL_6 = modified CL_6, that is, positive electrode on chest at C_6 (V_6) position with negative electrode at left shoulder.

H5 = Holter recording with positive electrode at C_5 (V_5) position.

When tracings consist of more than one strip, only the first strip is labeled if they form a continuous record. If the strips are not continuous, each strip is individually labeled.

RECOMMENDED READING

Fisch, C.: Electrocardiography of Arrhythmias. Philadelphia, Lea & Febiger, 1989.

Josephson, M.E., and Wellens, H.J.J.: Tachycardias: Mechanisms, Diagnosis, Treatment. Philadelphia, Lea & Febiger, 1984.

Kastor, J.A.: Arrhythmias. Philadelphia, W.B. Saunders, 1994.

Marriott, H.J.L.: Pearls and Pitfalls in Electrocardiography. Philadelphia, Lea & Febiger, 1990.

Marriott, H.J.L., and Conover, M.B.: Advanced Concepts in Arrhythmias. St. Louis, C.V. Mosby, 1983.

Pick, A., and Langendorf, R.: Interpretation of Complex Arrhythmias. Philadelphia, Lea & Febiger, 1979.

Wellens, H.J.J., and Kulbertus, H.E.: What's New in Electrocardiography? Boston, Martinus Nijhoff, 1981.

Wellens, H.J.J., and Conover, M.B.: The ECG in Emergency Decision Making. Philadelphia, W.B. Saunders, 1992.

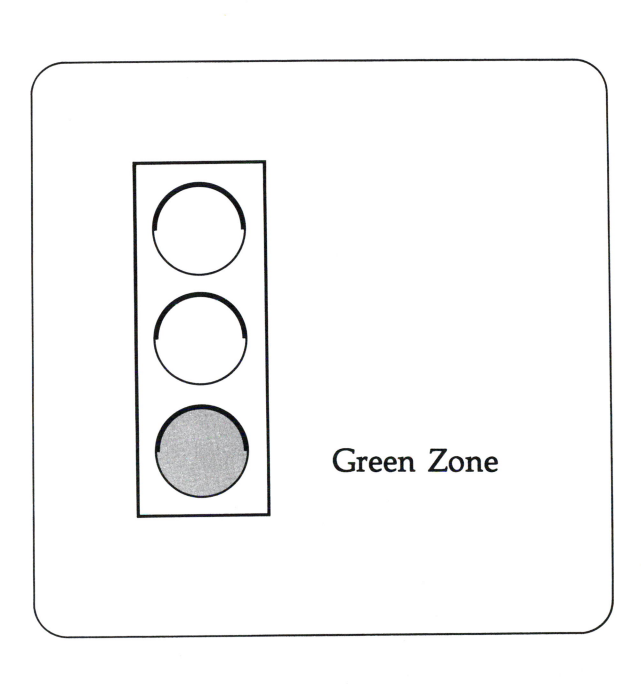

Green Zone

1

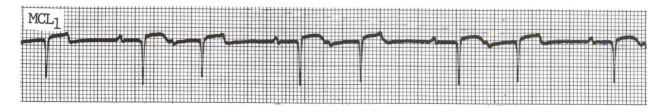

2

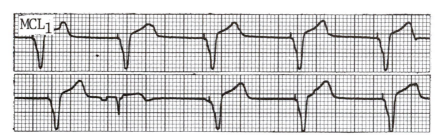

3

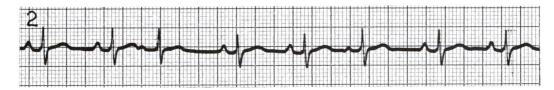

4

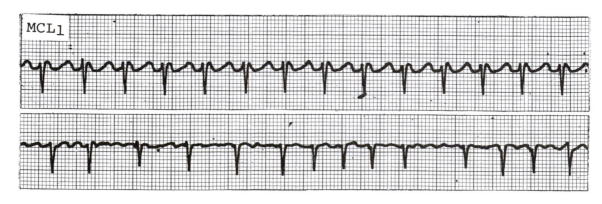

1

Diagnosis. **Sinus tachycardia** (rate 108/min) with **Type I A-V block** in the form of 3:2 **Wenckebach periods.** (The QRS-T configuration suggests anteroseptal infarction.)

2

Diagnosis. Right ventricular **demand pacemaker** at rate of 65/min.

Special Point. The pacemaker is identified as a demand model by the fact that it is inhibited by the natural (sinus) beat in the bottom strip.

3

Diagnosis. **Sinus rhythm at rate of 82/min, interrupted by two APBs** (third and sixth beats).

4

Diagnosis. Top strip: **atrial flutter** (rate 280/min) with 2:1 A-V conduction. Bottom strip: **atrial fibrillation** with rapid ventricular response (about 144/min).

Treatment. As usual, the primary goal of therapy is to *restore a normal ventricular rate*, and the secondary goal is to restore normal sinus rhythm.

Therefore, avoid quinidine (which is likely to accelerate the ventricular response) and use digitalis, verapamil, or propranolol until the ventricular rate is controlled; at that point, quinidine, procainamide, or a combination may be used to convert the arrhythmia. Countershock is, of course, an alternative that may achieve both goals simultaneously.

5

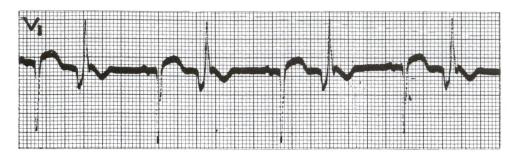

6

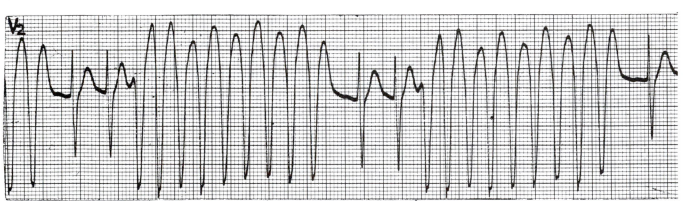

7

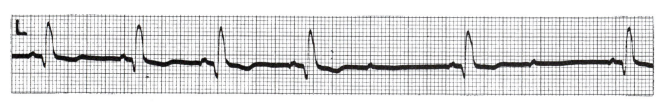

8

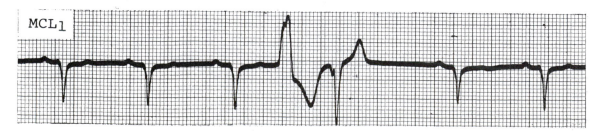

5

Diagnosis. Sinus rhythm with ventricular bigeminy.

Special Point. Note that the VPBs, with their wide Q waves, elevated ST segments, and inverted T waves, are even more diagnostic of the underlying anteroseptal infarction than is the pattern of the conducted ventricular complexes.[a]

Treatment. In the presence of an acute anterior infarction, the VPBs should be suppressed, if possible, with lidocaine.

[a] Bisteni, A., Medrano, G. A., and Sodi-Pallares, D.: Ventricular premature beats in the diagnosis of myocardial infarction. Br. Heart J. *23*:521, 1961.

6

Diagnosis. Paroxysms of repetitive ventricular tachycardia (rate 275/min) separated by pairs of sinus beats with rates of 150–160/min.

Special Point. This arrhythmia was seen in a 32-year-old nurse with an otherwise normal heart.

Treatment. Therapy consists of trial and error with antiarrhythmic agents such as quinidine, procainamide, tocainide, flecainide, disopyramide, mexiletine, and propranolol. If all else fails, amiodarone may be tried. Because the paroxysms are short and self-terminating, countershock has no place in therapy.

7

Diagnosis. Type II A-V block with LBBB. (The wide Q waves in aVL are virtually diagnostic of an anterior infarction, old or new.)

Special Point. The diagnosis of Type II block is made when *consecutive* atrial impulses are conducted with constant P-R intervals before the dropped beat. Note also that the combination of normal P-R intervals with bundle-branch block is characteristic of Type II block.

Treatment. Genuine Type II block invariably indicates a pacemaker.

8

Diagnosis. Sinus rhythm interrupted by a pair of bifocal VPBs.

Special Point. Judging by the polarity, the first VPB arises from the left ventricle and the second from the right.

9

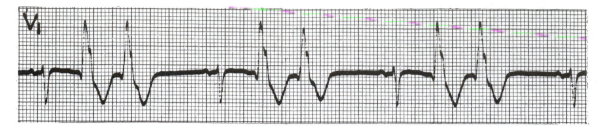

10

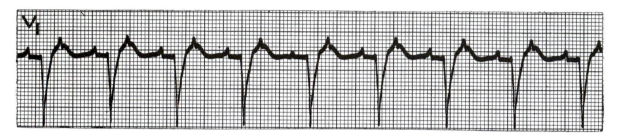

11

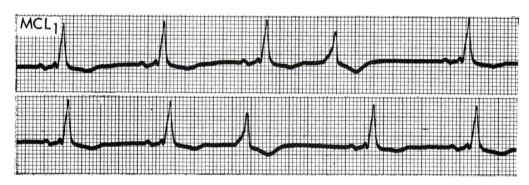

12

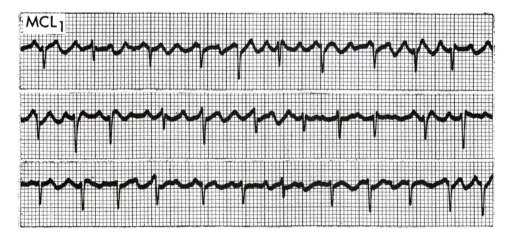

9

Diagnosis. **Sinus rhythm with paired left VPBs** producing ventricular "trigeminy."

Special Point. Note the typical QRS morphology: qR with taller left peak ("rabbit ear").

10

Diagnosis. **Atrial tachycardia** (rate 166/min) with 2:1 conduction and **LBBB.**

Special Points. Many clinicians do not have a cutoff rate above which they speak of 2:1 "conduction" and below which they pronounce 2:1 "block." Block implies abnormality, whereas conduction does not necessarily. Yet when atrial flutter is associated with 2:1 conduction, many call it 2:1 block, although it is clearly a normal function of the A-V node to prevent ventricles from following frenetic atria at a rate of 300/min.

My own arbitrary cutoff is 135/min. At an atrial rate above 135, I say 2:1 *conduction*; at an atrial rate under 135, I say 2:1 *block*.

It is impossible to tell in this tracing which P wave represents the conducted impulse—whether the P'-R interval is 0.16 or 0.50 sec.

11

Diagnosis. **Sinus bradycardia** (rate 54/min) with **RBBB; two left VPBs.**

Special Point. Note that in a right chest lead, such as V_1 or MCL_1, the main deflection of *right* bundle-branch block and of *left* VPBs is positive.

12

Diagnosis. **Coarse atrial fibrillation** with rapid ventricular response (rate about 125/min).

13

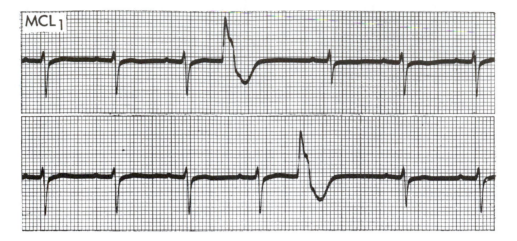

14

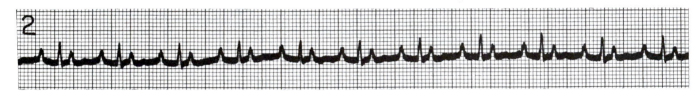

15

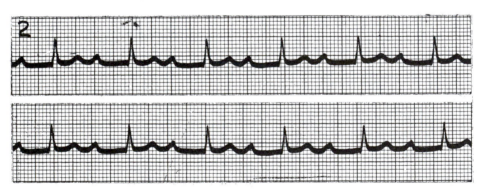

16

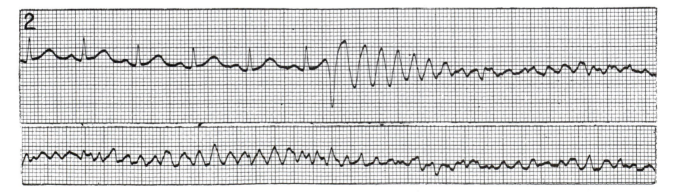

13

Diagnosis. Sinus rhythm interrupted by two left VPBs.

Special Point. Note the typical morphology of the VPBs, with early peak and slurring on the downstroke (taller left "rabbit-ear" equivalent).

14

Diagnosis. Atrial tachycardia (rate 190/min) with **2:1 A-V conduction.**

15

Diagnosis. First-degree A-V block. All atrial impulses are conducted with the same prolonged P-R interval (0.40 sec).

16

Diagnosis. Sinus rhythm interrupted by VPB, which precipitates ventricular fibrillation. (The tracing shows evidence of the underlying acute inferior infarction—slight ST elevation in lead 2.)

Special Points. The VPB interrupts the T wave of the sinus beat (R-on-T phenomenon).[a] Although there is no question that later VPBs can spark ventricular tachycardia or fibrillation, it is still probably true that a higher percentage of R-on-T extrasystoles will create that havoc.[b]

[a] Smirk, F. H., and Palmer, D. G.: A myocarcardial syndrome, with particular reference to the occurrence of sudden death and of premature systoles interrupting antecedent T waves. Am. J. Cardiol. 6:620, 1960.
[b] Adgey, A. A. J., Devlin, J. E., Webb, S. W., and Mulholland, H. C.: Initiation of ventricular fibrillation outside hospital in patients with ischemic heart disease. Br. Heart J. 47:55, 1982.

17

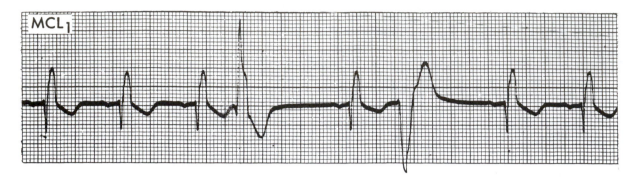

18

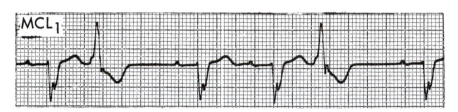

19

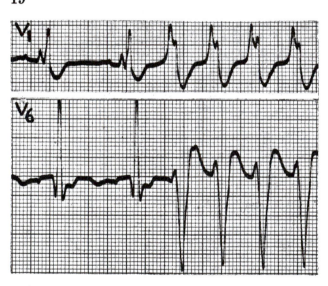

20

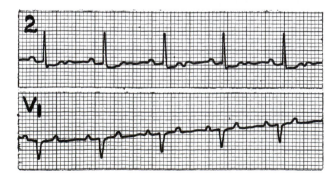

17

Diagnosis. **Sinus rhythm with RBBB** interrupted by first a **left** and then a presumably **right VPB.**

Special Point. The morphology of the left VPB is virtually diagnostic, with its steep upstroke, early peak, and slurring on the downstroke (taller left rabbit-ear equivalent).

18

Diagnosis. **Sinus rhythm with first-degree A-V block** and **LBBB;** two left **VPBs.**

19

Diagnosis. **Sinus rhythm with RBBB** interrupted by bursts of **left ventricular tachycardia** (rate 140/min).

Special Point. Note the typical morphology of RBBB (rsR´ in V_1 and qRs in V_6) and of left ventricular ectopy (monophasic R with taller left rabbit ear in V_1,[a] with absent Q, small R, and deeper, wider S wave—more than 15 mm deep—in V_6).

[a] Gozensky, C., and Thorne, D: Rabbit ears: an aid in distinguishing ventricular ectopy from aberration. Heart Lung 3:634, 1974.

20

Diagnosis. **Atrial tachycardia** (rate 186/min) with **2:1 A-V conduction.**

21

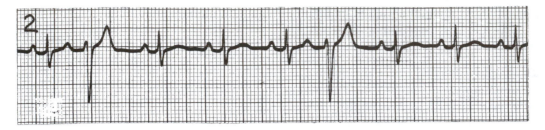

22

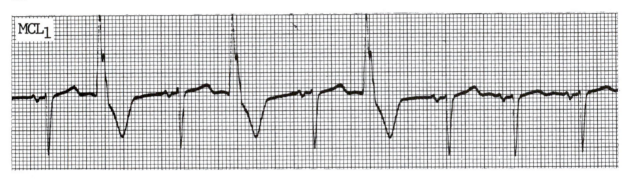

23

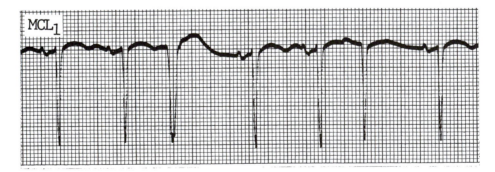

21

Diagnosis. Sinus rhythm at rate of 88/min interrupted by two APBs conducted with **ventricular aberration.**

Special Points. The axis shift in the aberrant beats probably identifies it as left anterior hemiblock aberration; the premature P waves preceding each aberrant QRS are identified by the slight apparent sharpening and increased height of the T waves.

22

Diagnosis. Sinus rhythm interrupted by a run of left ventricular bigeminy.

Special Point. Note the characteristic morphology for left ventricular ectopy: tall, early peak with notching on the downstroke.

23

Diagnosis. Sinus rhythm interrupted by first a right VPB and then an APB. (The depth of this S wave in MCL_1 is consistent with left ventricular hypertrophy.)

Special Point. Note that the VPB is followed by a fully compensatory pause, whereas the APB is not—136 equals two sinus cycles (68×2), and 127 does not.

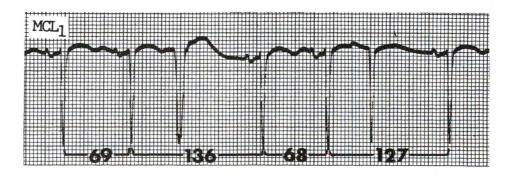

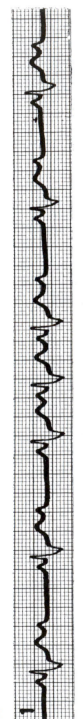

24

1

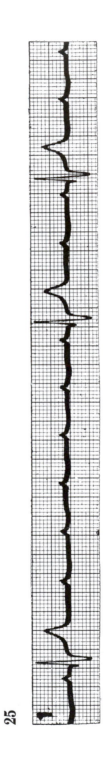

25

1

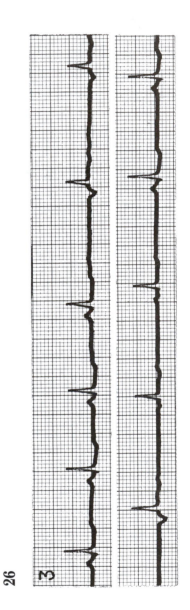

26

3

24

Diagnosis. Sinus rhythm (rate 98/min) with 1:1 A-V conduction and Type II 2:1 A-V block; RBBB.

Special Point. The unchanging and normal P-R interval in the *consecutively* conducted beats (before the next dropped beat) firmly establishes the diagnosis of Type II block.

25

Diagnosis. High grade A-V block, presumably Type II, with **RBBB.**

Special Point. The combination of normal P-R interval with BBB and the series of several *consecutive* blocked atrial impulses are characteristic of Type II block.

High grade A-V block is diagnosed when two or more than two consecutive atrial impulses, at a reasonable atrial rate (<135/min), fail to be conducted *because of the block itself.* (Compare with other later tracings in which most atrial impulses are not conducted, yet the block itself is mild—see Figures 150, 164, 170, and 173.)

26

Diagnosis. Shifting (or wandering) **pacemaker.** After four sinus beats, the sinus pause ends with atrial (or junctional) escape for three beats. In the bottom strip, the last two beats are again sinus, whereas the second and third beats probably represent **atrial fusion.**

27

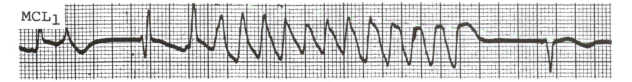

28

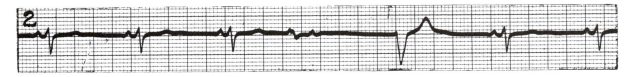

29

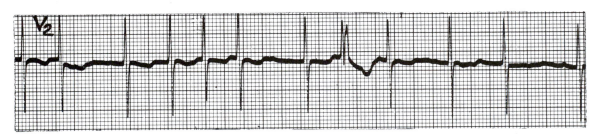

30

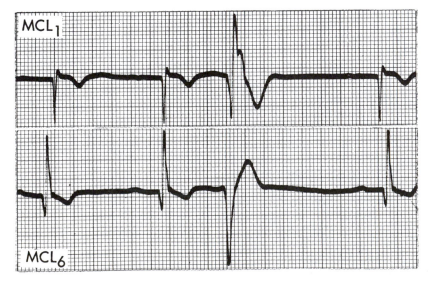

27

Diagnosis. **Torsades de pointes**—"twistings of the points."

Special Point. After two or three nondescript ventricular complexes, a short paroxysm of torsades develops in which the points twist from positive to negative. Note the prolonged Q-T interval in the beat before and after the paroxysm.

28

Diagnosis. **Sinus rhythm interrupted by a VPB;** the postextrasystolic cycle ends with a **ventricular escape** beat.

29

Diagnosis. **Atrial fibrillation** with moderately rapid ventricular response (112/min); one **aberrantly conducted** beat.

Special Point. Note that the relatively long cycle followed by a relatively short cycle precipitates the RBBB aberration (Ashman phenomenon).[a]

Treatment. Restore a normal ventricular rate with digitalis, verapamil, propranolol, or cardioversion.

[a] Gouaux, J. L., and Ashman, R.: Auricular fibrillation with aberration simulating ventricular paroxysmal tachycardia. Am. Heart J. *34*:366, 1947.

30

Diagnosis. **Sinus bradycardia** (49/min) with **first-degree A-V block** (P-R = 0.32 sec); **VPBs.** (The QRS pattern in both leads suggests anterior myocardial infarction.)

Special Point. The QR pattern in MCL_1 with the taller left peak is characteristic of left ventricular ectopy, as is the rS pattern in MCL_6, especially with an S wave 20 mm deep.

Treatment. Atropine judiciously administered to increase the cardiac rate may also eliminate the ventricular ectopy.

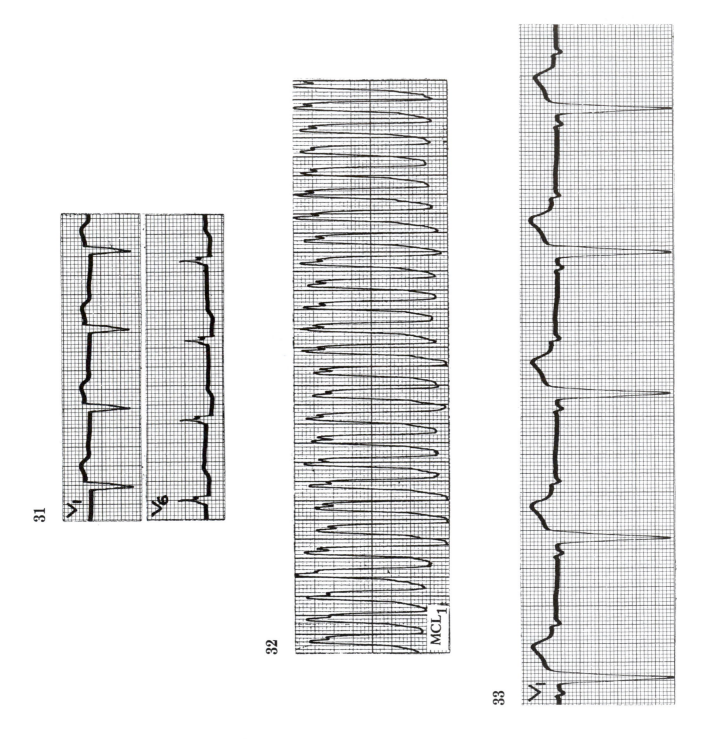

31

32

33

31

Diagnosis. Accelerated junctional rhythm (rate 74/min) with **incomplete LBBB.**

Special Point. Early signs of LBBB are slight widening of QRS with loss of r in V_1 and loss of q in V_6.

32

Diagnosis. Left ventricular tachycardia (rate 260/min).

Special Point. The taller left rabbit ear identifies the rhythm as ectopic ventricular rather than supraventricular with aberration. This pattern can, however, be a supraventricular tachycardia with Wolff-Parkinson-White conduction.

Treatment. Prompt termination with low dosage (10–20 joules) electrical cardioversion. A bolus of lidocaine (50–75 mg) given intravenously may be tried while awaiting the cardioverter.

33

Diagnosis. 2:1 A-V block, probably Type II; **LBBB.**

Special Point. The combination of a normal P-R interval with a bundle-branch block makes a Type II (bilateral BBB) A-V block likely.

Treatment. If Type II block is confirmed, a permanent pacemaker is indicated.

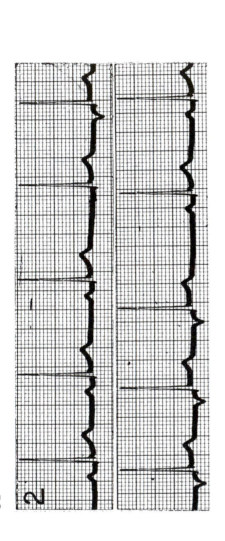

34

2

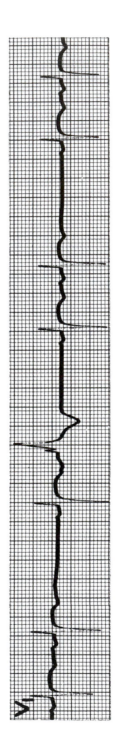

35

V₁

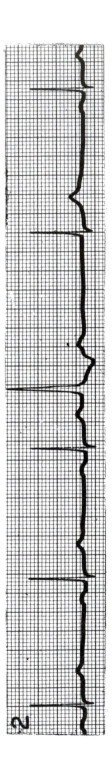

36

2

34

cycle lengthens and the next descending impulse meets the retrograde impulse from the awakening junction to produce atrial fusion. The junction maintains control for the next four beats and then slows and permits the sinus rhythm to again take over.

Diagnosis. **Shifting** (or wandering) **pacemaker; atrial fusion.**

Special Point. In a typical shifting pacemaker, the shift occurs only when one pacemaker slows and permits the other to escape. In this tracing, after three regular sinus beats, the sinus

35

Treatment. APBs generally require no treatment; if they are frequent and troublesome, they may be suppressed by any number of antiarrhythmic agents such as quinidine, digoxin, or propranolol. Sometimes they are a sign of early congestive heart failure, and then digoxin is the obvious choice.

Diagnosis. **Sinus rhythm with atrial bigeminy,** with the second APB showing **RBBB aberration.**

Special Point. The reason only the second APB is conducted aberrantly is because it is more premature than the other three and consequently ends a shorter ventricular cycle.

36

Diagnosis. **Sinus bradycardia** (rate 48/min); **intraatrial block; first-degree A-V block** (P-R = 0.25 sec); **VPB; junctional escape.**

Treatment. No treatment is required unless the slow rate is causing symptoms; if so, treat as for sick sinus syndrome.

37

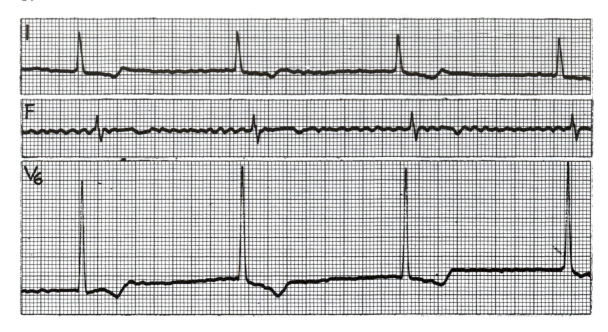

38

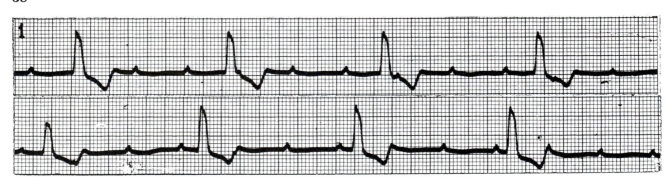

39

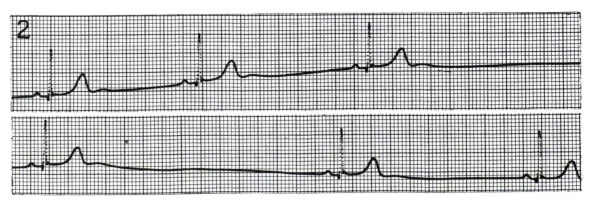

37

Diagnosis. **Atrial fibrillation** with **complete A-V block** and **junctional escape** rhythm (rate = 35/min).

Special Point. Because of the atrial fibrillation, the block may not be as bad as it looks, because concealed conduction into the junction is superimposed on the block and the effect of its contribution cannot be evaluated. The block might turn out to be comparatively minor if sinus rhythm was restored.

However, this patient may indeed need a pacemaker, avoiding atrial fibrillation. But one should keep in mind that because of the concealed conduction that invariably accompanies atrial flutter and fibrillation, the block usually appears worse than it is. For instance, if sinus rhythm could be maintained, the heart of a patient such as this might be perfectly capable of conducting every beat at a normal sinus rate.

Treatment. The patient should first be cardioverted to assess the degree of block during sinus rhythm and should then be treated accordingly.

38

Diagnosis. Sinus tachycardia (rate 106/min) with **complete A-V block** and **idioventricular rhythm** at a rate of 36/min.

Special Point. This has all the criteria for a diagnosis of complete A-V block: (1) no conduction, in the presence of (2) a slow enough ventricular rate (under 45/min) and (3) P waves that march across the R-R interval, probing all phases of the ventricular cycle.

Treatment. Genuine complete A-V block, such as this, almost always requires a permanent artificial pacemaker.

39

Diagnosis. Sick sinus syndrome manifested by an extreme and irregular sinus bradycardia.

Special Point. It is of course impossible to pinpoint the mechanism in such cases, that is, whether the sinus bradycardia is due to sluggish and erratic behavior on the part of the sinus pacemaking mechanism or to exit block out of the sinus node. The general rule is if one can establish a mathematical relationship between the cycle lengths, one can diagnose exit block; if there is no such discernible relationship, one attributes the bradyarrhythmia to "generator failure."

40

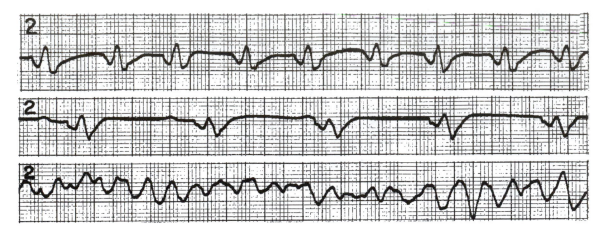

41

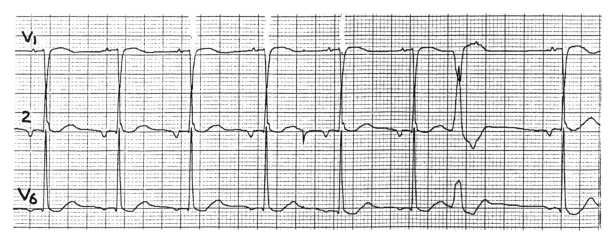

40

Diagnosis. **Agonal rhythm** slowing and degenerating into **ventricular fibrillation.**

Special Point. Agonal rhythm is a terminal, ineffectual rhythm, so named from the Greek agōn, meaning struggle.

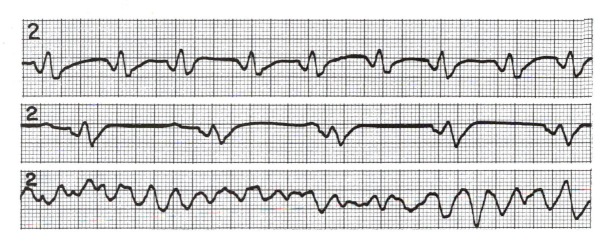

41

Diagnosis. **Ectopic atrial rhythm** (inverted P waves in 2 and V$_6$ with normal P-R interval) interrupted by a single **VPB**, presumably from the right ventricle (LBBB pattern).

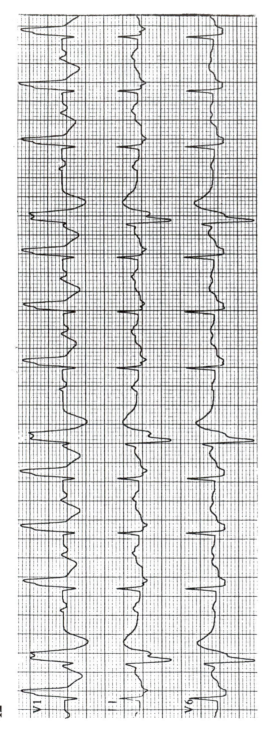

42

V1

I

V2

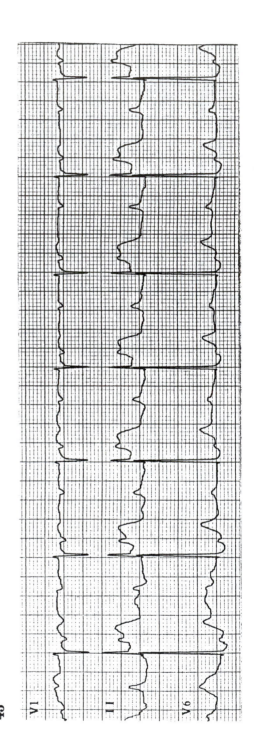

43

V1

II

V6

42

Diagnosis. Sinus tachycardia with first-degree A-V block (P-R = 0.22 sec) and **RBBB** interrupted by **left VPBs** every fourth beat.

43

Diagnosis. Sinus tachycardia (rate 120/min), with **2:1, Type I, second-degree A-V block** (in patient with acute inferior myocardial infarction).

44

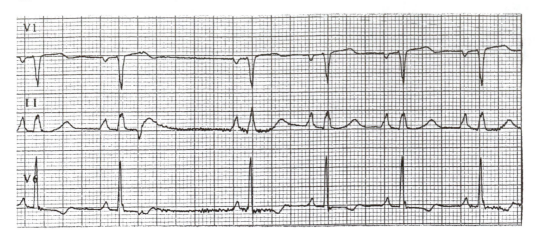

45

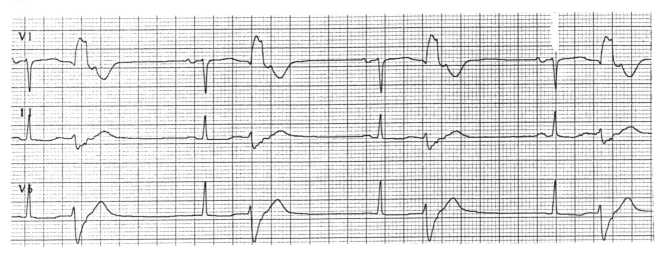

44

Diagnosis. Sinus rhythm interrupted by a **nonconducted APB**. (P waves suggest biatrial hypertrophy).

45

Diagnosis. Sinus rhythm with left ventricular bigeminy with retrograde conduction to atria.

Special point. Note typical morphology of left ventricular ectopy—taller left rabbit ear in V_1 with absent q and rS in V_6.

46

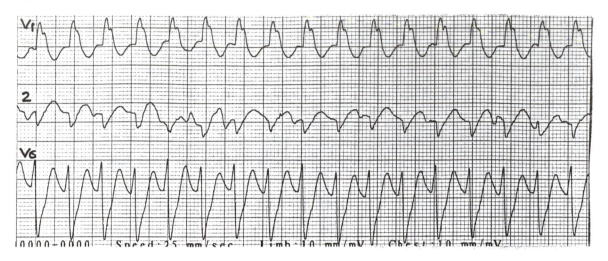

47

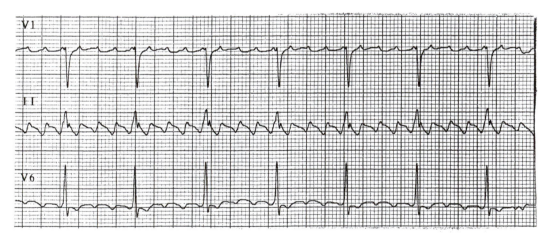

46

Diagnosis. Left ventricular tachycardia (rate 170/min).

Special Point. Note taller left rabbit ear in V_1, absent Q with RS ratio less than 1 in V_6, and 2 : 1 and 3 : 1 retrograde conduction to the atria (well seen in lead 2—see laddergram).

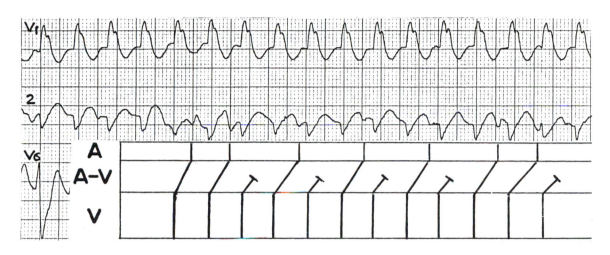

47

Diagnosis. **Atrial flutter** with 4 : 1 A-V conduction.

Special Point. Note the characteristic morphology of the atrial waves: typical "saw-toothed" or "picket-fence" pattern in the inferior lead (lead 2), with upright P-like waves in V_1 and inverted P-like waves in V_6.

48

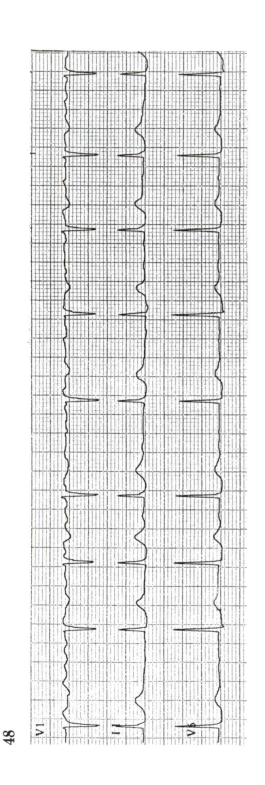

V1

II

V6

49

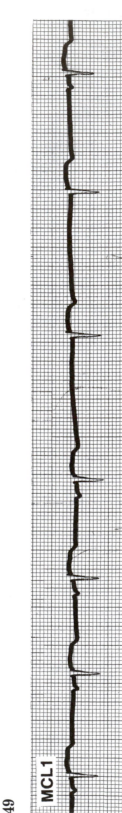

MCL1

50

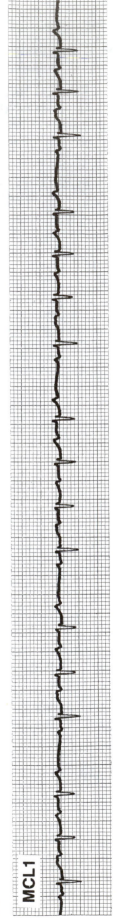

MCL1

48

Diagnosis. Atrial fibrillation with controlled ventricular response.

49

Diagnosis. Sinus bradycardia interrupted by a prolonged **sinus pause** providing the opportunity for two consecutive **junctional escape beats.**

50

Diagnosis. Sinus tachycardia (rate 135/min) with 4:3 and 5:4 **A-V Wenckebach periods.**

51

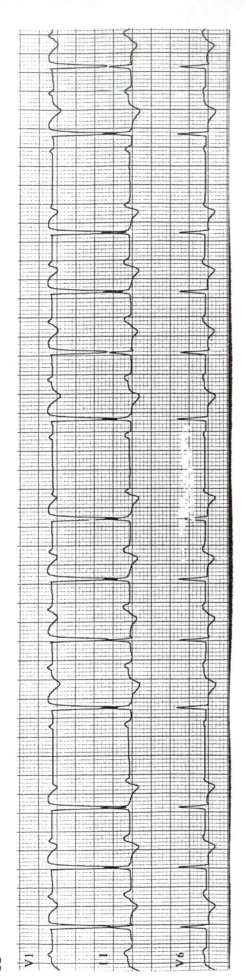

V1

II

V6

52

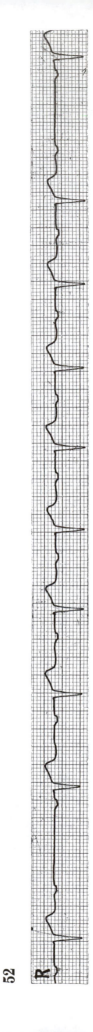

R

51

Diagnosis. Sinus rhythm (rate 96/min) with 5:4 A-V Wenckebach periods.

52

Diagnosis. Sinus rhythm with **9:8 A-V Wenckebach periods.**

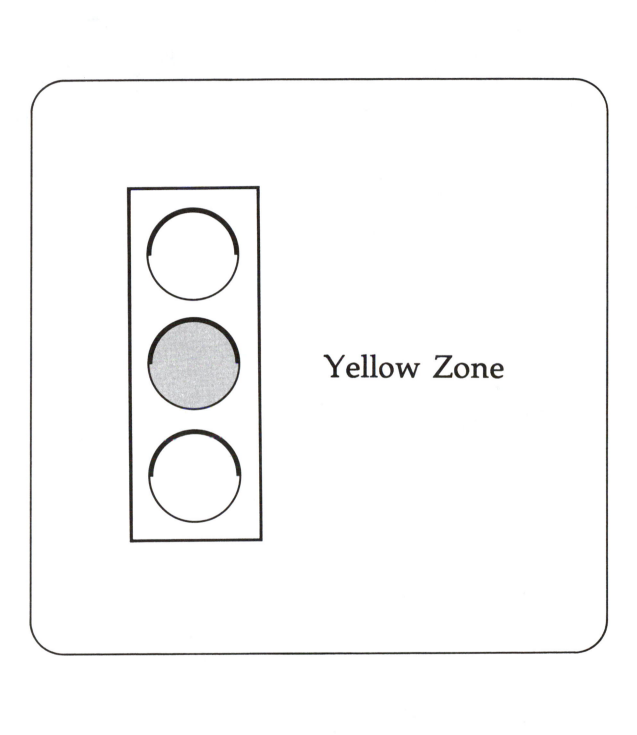

Yellow Zone

53

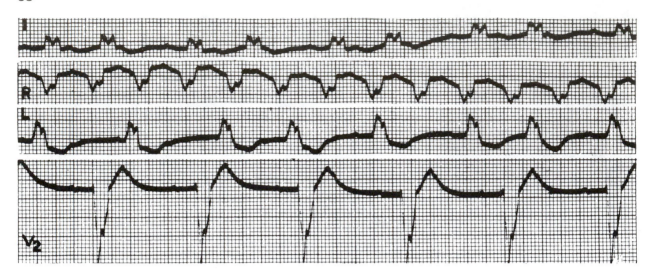

54

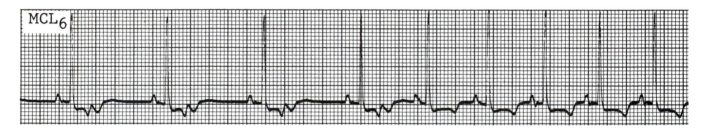

55

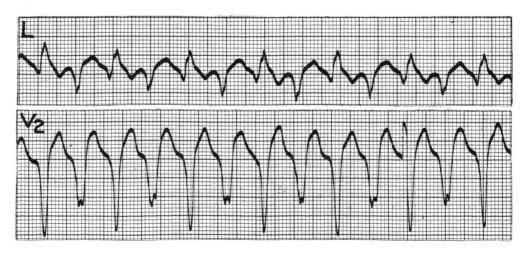

53

Diagnosis. **Sinus tachycardia** (rate 110/min); **Type I A-V block** with 3:2 Wenckebach periods in lead 1, 1:1 conduction in aVR, 2:1 and 3:1 conduction in aVL, and 2:1 conduction in V_2; **LBBB.**

54

Diagnosis. **Sinus rhythm with nonconducted atrial bigeminy** followed by **sinus tachycardia.** (The QRS-T pattern is typical of left ventricular hypertrophy.)

55

Diagnosis. **Bidirectional** (top strip) and **alternating** (bottom strip) patterns of **ventricular tachycardia.**

Special Point. Note that "bidirectional" and "alternating" are purely descriptive of the patterns seen in the leads you happen to be looking at. Neither term identifies a specific form of VT. Some of these tachycardias may indeed be ectopic ventricular with alternating sequences of ventricular activation. Some may be due to junctional tachycardia with RBBB and alternating hemiblocks.[a]

[a] Cohen, S. I., and Voukydis, P.: Supraventricular origin of bidirectional tachycardia. Circulation *50*:634, 1974.

56

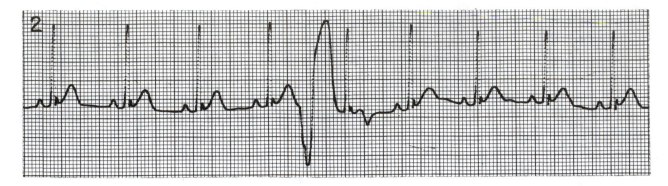

57

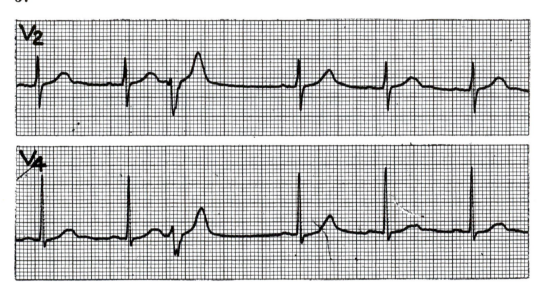

58

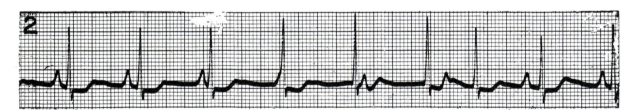

56

Diagnosis. **Sinus rhythm interrupted by an interpolated VPB.**

Special Point. Note that the T wave of the sinus beat after the VPB is inverted. This does not have the same unfavorable significance as the usual "postextrasystolic T-wave change" in the beat ending a compensatory pause (see Figure 45). Rather, this is a form of aberration, affecting only the T wave, which results from an abrupt shortening of the cycle.

57

Diagnosis. **VPBs** followed by fully compensatory pauses and postextrasystolic T-wave changes.

Special Point. A change in the T wave of the sinus beat ending a compensatory pause after a VPB is suspicious, although not diagnostic, of myocardial disease.[a]

[a] Leachman, D. R., Dehmer, G. J., Firth, B. G., Markham, R. V., Jr., Winniford, M. D., and Hillis, L. D.: Evaluation of postextrasystolic T wave alterations in identification of patients with coronary artery disease or left ventricular dysfunction. Am. Heart J. *102*:658, 1981.

58

Diagnosis. **Accelerated idiojunctional rhythm** (rate 76/min) producing **A-V dissociation** with two **ventricular captures,** the first conducted with prolonged P-R interval (see laddergram).

Special Point. This arrhythmia was caused by digitalis intoxication in a 10-year-old girl who had recently required a valvotomy for tight mitral stenosis.

Treatment. Discontinue digitalis.

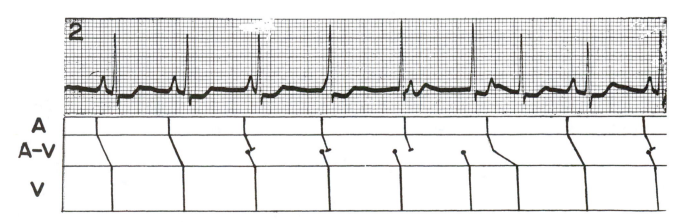

59

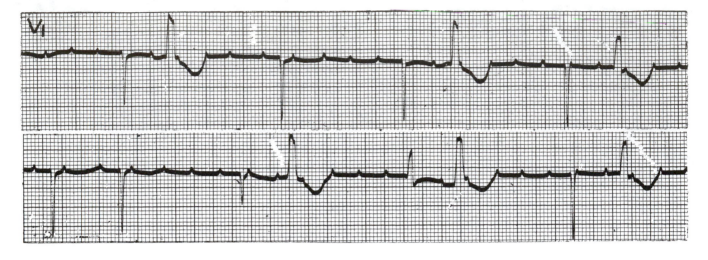

60

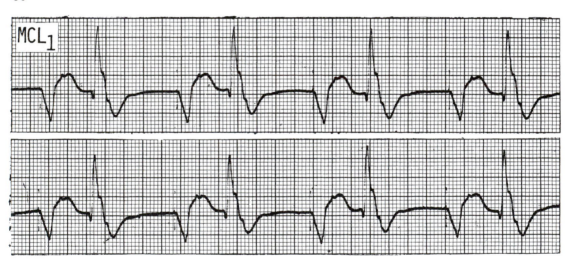

61

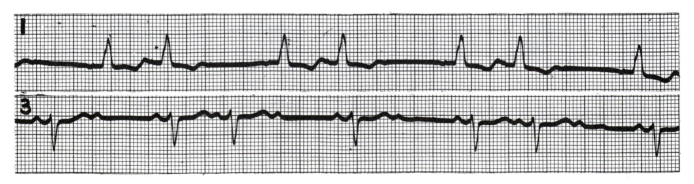

59

Diagnosis. **Atrial tachycardia** (rate 205/min) with varying A-V block and frequent **left ventricular extrasystoles.** The third beat in the lower strip is probably a **junctional escape** beat, and the fifth beat is probably a **ventricular escape.**

Special Point. The P waves of atrial tachycardia caused by digitalis intoxication are usually normally directed, smaller than average, and somewhat irregular. This arrhythmia developed postpartum in a 32-year-old woman with puerperal cardiomyopathy who developed congestive failure and was mistakenly digitalized with 2 mg of digoxin intravenously.

60

Diagnosis. **Artificial right ventricular pacemaker** with retrograde conduction to the atria; **left ventricular bigeminy.**

Special Point. At first inspection, in view of the retrograde conduction, one might believe the second beat in each pair was a reciprocal beat with RBBB aberration. Against this is the QRS morphology and the R-P:P-R ratio. The second QRS complex, unlike RBBB, has an early peak with slurring on the downstroke (taller left rabbit ear equivalent) and the R-P is shorter than the P-R, whereas with reciprocal beating, the R-P is almost always longer than the P-R (as in Figure 169).

61

Diagnosis. **3:2 and 2:1 Type II A-V block; LBBB.**

Special Points. This is typical in every way of Type II A-V block: not only is the P-R interval constant in consecutive beats preceding dropped beats, but the other two classic features—normal P-R and BBB—are also evident.

62

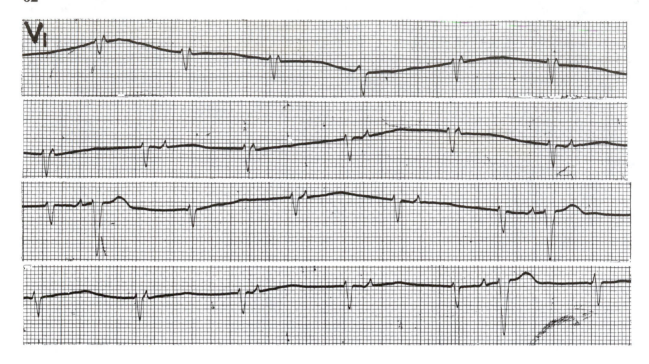

63

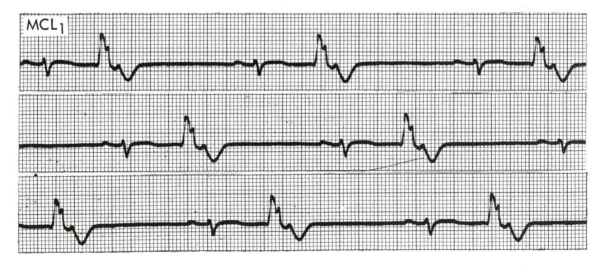

62

Diagnosis. **Sinus bradycardia** with resulting **junctional escape** and **A-V dissociation**; three **ventricular captures** with **LBBB aberration**.

Special Points. Note that both sinus and junctional rhythms are somewhat irregular. The junctional rhythm starts off at an accelerated rate of about 65/min and then slows to about 54/min.

The only primary diagnoses are the sinus bradycardia and the rate-dependent LBBB; escape, dissociation, and capture are all secondary to the sinus bradycardia.

63

Diagnosis. **Sinus bradycardia** with borderline P-R interval (0.20 sec) and **left ventricular bigeminy with** retrograde conduction to the atria (arrows).

Special Point. Retrograde conduction to the atria after ventricular premature beats is common,[a] and the normal R-P interval after such beats is the same as the normal P-R interval, that is, 0.12–0.20 sec.

[a] Kistin, A., and Landowne, M.: Retrograde conduction from premature ventricular contractions, a common occurrence in the human heart. Circulation *3*:738, 1951.

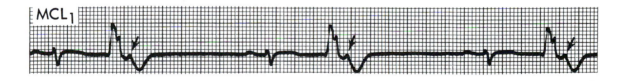

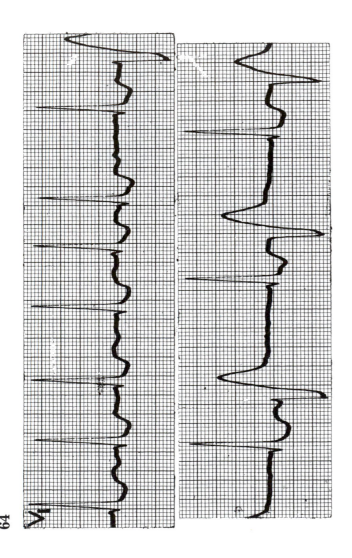

64

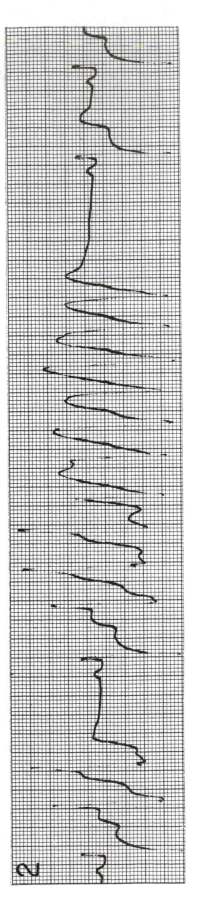

65

64

Diagnosis. **Atrial fibrillation** with moderate ventricular response (about 88/min). Toward the end of the top strip, lengthening of the ventricular cycle precipitates **right ventricular bigeminy.**

Special Point. The "rule of bigeminy"[b] is that a lengthened ventricular cycle tends to precipitate a ventricular extrasystole and that the resulting ventricular ectopy tends to be self-perpetuating, because each ventricular extrasystole is in turn followed by a lengthened cycle.

[b] Langendorf, R., Pick, A., and Winternitz, M.: Mechanisms of intermittent ventricular bigeminy. I. Appearance of ectopic beats dependent upon the length of the ventricular cycle, the "rule of bigeminy." Circulation *11*:442, 1955.

65

Diagnosis. **Torsades de pointes** (twistings of the points) from a patient during a paroxysm of variant angina.

Special Points. Note that the apices of the ectopic beats first point upward and then downward; this form of twisting is characteristic of torsades. Notice the marked ST segment depression in the sinus beats, signifying the severe ischemia. The QT interval of the sinus beats is prolonged, another characteristic of torsades.

Treatment. The first step in treating torsades is to eliminate any curable cause. This includes withholding antiarrhythmic agents, phenothiazines, and tricyclic antidepressants; correcting hypokalemia and hypomagnesemia; and accelerating a bradycardia. Drugs that may be successful are isoproterenol (which shortens the QT interval), potassium, magnesium, and mexiletine (which does not lengthen the QT interval). A temporary pacemaker, programed at 100+/min, may be needed to control the situation.

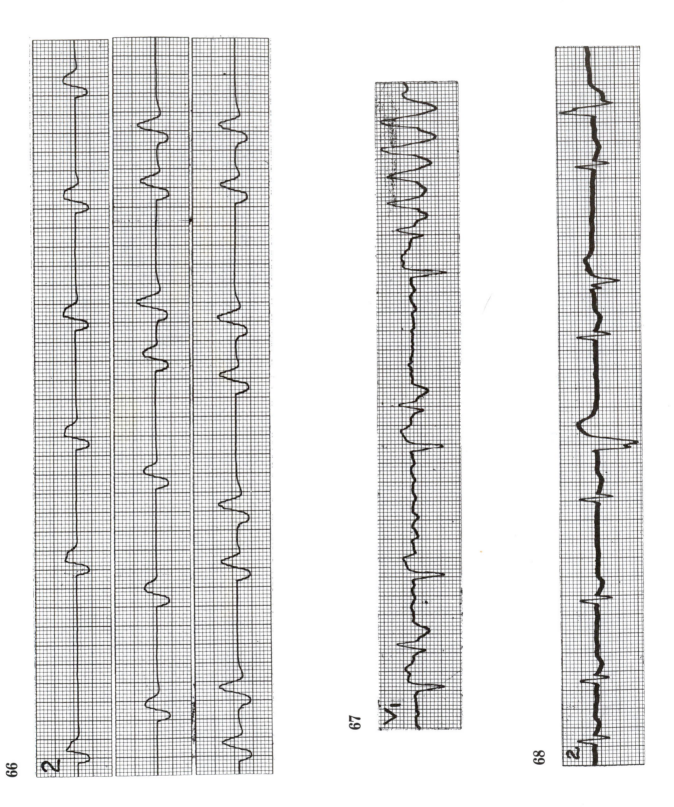

66

Diagnosis. Agonal rhythm.

Special Points. These bizarre, grossly widened complexes are typical of agonal rhythm. In such terminal throes, there is usually no atrial activity and the ventricular complexes may be quite irregular.

67

Diagnosis. Atrial fibrillation with slow ventricular response; **ventricular extrasystoles**, the third of which precipitates **left ventricular tachycardia.**

Special Points. During atrial fibrillation, it may be particularly difficult to differentiate aberration from ectopy; here note the fixed coupling of the beats in question—a strong point in favor of ectopy.

A minor point in terminology: during atrial fibrillation, when one never knows when the next impulse will be conducted, the term *premature* beat is meaningless, and it is therefore more logical to use extrasystoles for beats with fixed coupling.

68

Diagnosis. Atrial fibrillation with moderate ventricular response and **multifocal ventricular extrasystoles** producing a run of **bigeminy.** (From a patient with digitalis intoxication.)

Special Point. When digitalis causes frequent ventricular extrasystoles, they are almost invariably multifocal.[a] Note the sagging ST segments of digitalis effect.

[a] Scherf, D., and Schott, A.: Extrasystoles and allied arrhythmias. 2nd Ed. New York, Grune & Stratton, 1973, pp. 586–587.

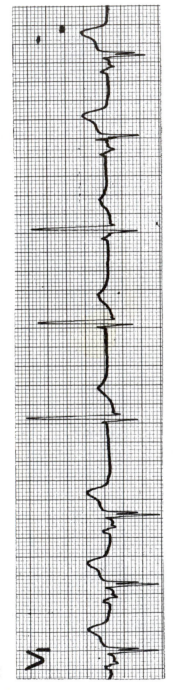

69

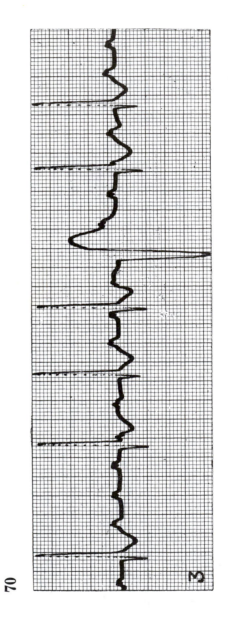

70

3

69

Diagnosis. After three sinus beats at a rate of 82/min, a sinus pause permits an **accelerated idioventricular rhythm** to escape for three beats at a rate of 60/min. The sinus node then accelerates and resumes control.

70

Diagnosis. Atrial tachycardia with varying **A-V block;** one **VPB.**

Special Point. From the tracing, one cannot be sure the arrhythmia is due to digitalis intoxication, but the sagging ST segments and short QT interval are certainly suggestive. Also, in the atrial tachycardia of digitalis intoxication, the P waves are usually, as these are, normally directed.

Treatment. In most such cases it is sufficient to discontinue the digitalis preparation and let the toxic effect abate. Available active treatments for digitalis intoxication include potassium, propranolol, phenytoin, and fab fragments.

71

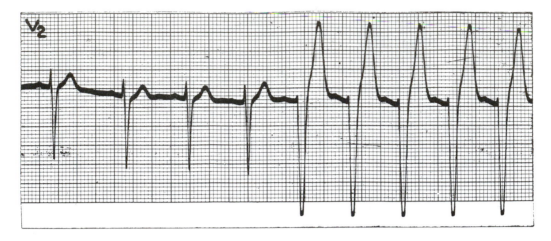

72

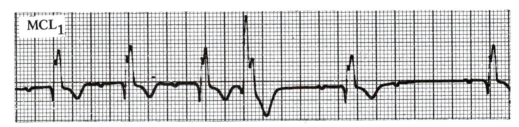

73

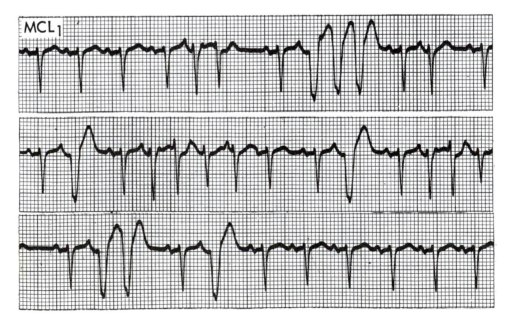

71

Diagnosis. **Sinus rhythm accelerating to sinus tachycardia** with development of **rate-dependent LBBB.**

Treatment. Bundle-branch block, whether dependent on rate or not, has no treatment. The cause of the accelerating sinus rate may require investigation and therapy.

72

Diagnosis. **Sinus rhythm with first-degree A-V block** (P-R = 0.29 sec) and **RBBB; VPB,** followed by **2:1 A-V block.**

Special Points. The qR pattern of the RBBB is suspicious of an underlying anteroseptal infarction. After the VPB, a 2:1 A-V ratio develops; this is because the longer cycle after the VPB lengthens the ensuing refractory period of the ventricular conduction system, so that the next, otherwise conductible, sinus impulse is blocked.

73

Diagnosis. **Sinus tachycardia** (rate 135/min) interrupted by **APBs,** with and without **LBBB aberration.** The salvos of three and five consecutive APBs qualify as short runs of ectopic **atrial tachycardia.**

74

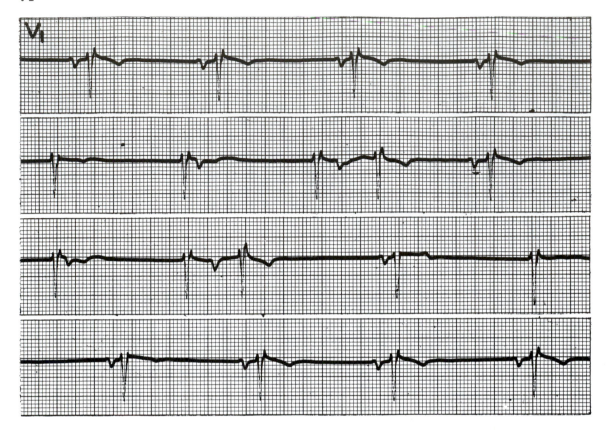

75

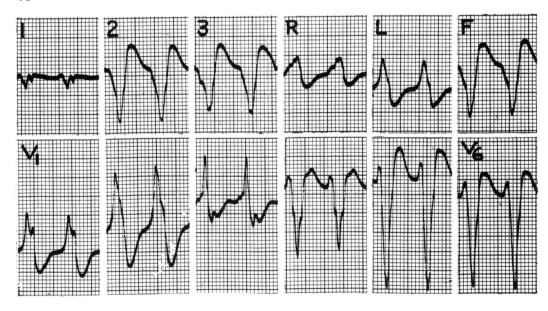

74

Diagnosis. Binodal disease: sinus bradycardia with arrhythmia. When the sinus rhythm slows to about 40/min, the junction takes over with a slightly faster rate, producing **A-V dissociation.** The early beats are **ventricular captures** with prolonged P-R intervals. Almost all QRS complexes show a pattern of **incomplete RBBB.**

Special Point. Note the reciprocal relationship between R-P and P-R in the two ventricular capture beats; this indicates the potential for Wenckebach-type conduction and signals A-V nodal disease. (The tracing is from a boy with congenital heart disease after surgery for ostium primum atrial septal defect with cleft mitral valve.) Note that the longest cycle in the third strip represents a rate of only 33/min.

75

Diagnosis. Each lead contains a sinus beat followed by a right ventricular extrasystole.

Special Point. These VPBs have the morphological features described by Rosenbaum[a] as characteristic of healthy subjects: an LBBB pattern in V_6, with two features elsewhere in the tracing that are quite unlike LBBB, namely, a fat little r wave in V_1 and a vertical or right axis deviation in the frontal plane. (This tracing was from an 18-year-old professional baseball pitcher.)

[a] Rosenbaum, M. B.: Classification of extrasystoles according to form. J. Electrocardiol. *2*:289, 1969.

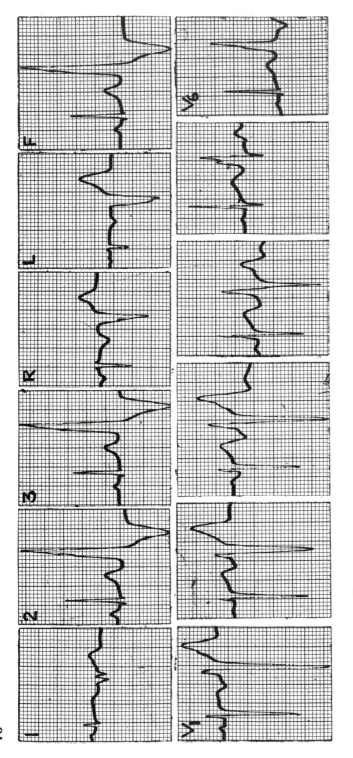

76

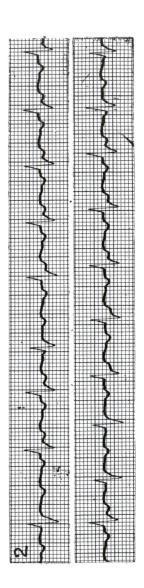

77

76

Diagnosis. **Left ventricular tachycardia.**

Special Point. This tracing shows four of the morphological features most characteristic of left ventricular ectopy: dominant R wave in V_1 with left peak taller than right (taller left rabbit ear); little R, deeper, wider S wave in V_6; negative deflection in V_6 deeper than 15 mm; and frontal plane axis in right upper quadrant ("no-man's land").

Ignorance or neglect of these and other morphological clues to ventricular ectopy has led to repeated errors in the diagnosis of wide QRS tachycardias. Recent publications[a-c] have documented a remarkable tendency to favor the diagnosis of supraventricular tachycardia with aberration when the QRS morphology strongly indicated the likelihood of ventricular ectopy. Study Figures 70, 104, 146, and 162 for additional important clues.

[a] Dancy, M., Camm, A. J., and Ward, D.: Misdiagnosis of chronic recurrent ventricular tachycardia. Lancet 2:320, 1985.
[b] Morady, F., Baerman, J. M., DiCarlo, L. A., and DeBuitleir, M.: A prevalent misconception regarding wide-complex tachycardias. JAMA 254:2790, 1985.
[c] Stewart, R. B., Bardy, G. H., and Greene, H. L.: Wide complex tachycardia: misdiagnosis and outcome after emergent therapy. Ann. Intern. Med. 104:766, 1986.

77

Diagnosis. **Atrial tachycardia** (rate 202/min) with varying A-V conduction, mostly 2:1.

Special Point. The fact that all atrial impulses are not conducted establishes the probability of ectopic (automatic) atrial tachycardia.[a]

[a] Bär, F. W., Brugada, P., Dassen, W. R., and Wellens, H. J.: Differential diagnosis of tachycardia with narrow QRS complex (shorter than 0.12 sec). Am. J. Cardiol. 54:555, 1984.

78

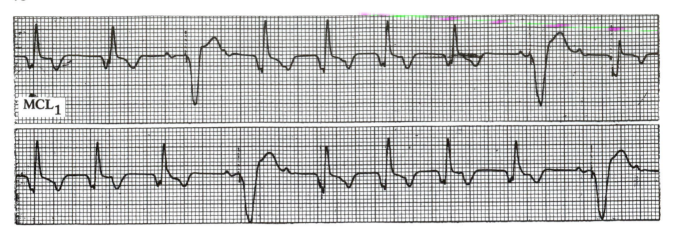

MCL$_1$

79

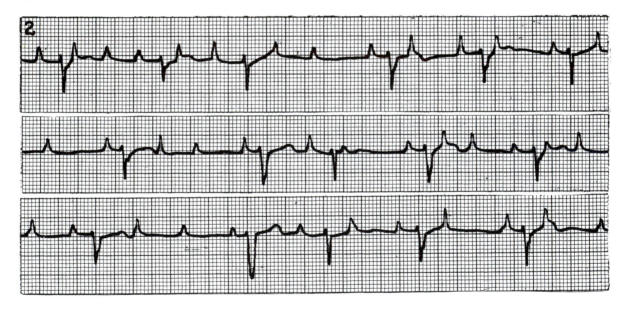

78

Diagnosis. **Sinus rhythm with Type I A-V block** (5:4 **Wenckebach periods**) with **RBBB;** right ventricular **demand pacemaker.** The third and last beats in the top strip are **fusion beats.** (Note the wide Q waves in the conducted beats, indicating the associated anterior infarction.)

Special Point. The P waves of the conducted beats during the Wenckebach period are difficult to identify because they land on the ST segment or T wave of the preceding beat. The dropped beat of each Wenckebach period provides a pause that permits the demand pacemaker to escape for one or two beats.

79

Diagnosis. **Multifocal** (or chaotic) **atrial tachycardia** with varying **A-V block** (from a patient with severe emphysema).

Special Point. Note that the P waves, although ectopic, bear the pointed, prominent stamp of P-pulmonale. Beats ending the longest cycles may be junctional or ventricular escapes. Note the marked axis shift indicated by the predominantly negative QRS complex in lead 2. Instead of the expected vertical axis, a minority of patients with chronic cor pulmonale have marked *left* axis deviation.

80

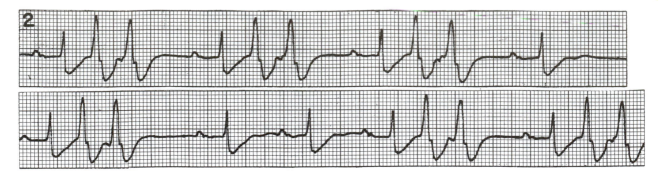

81

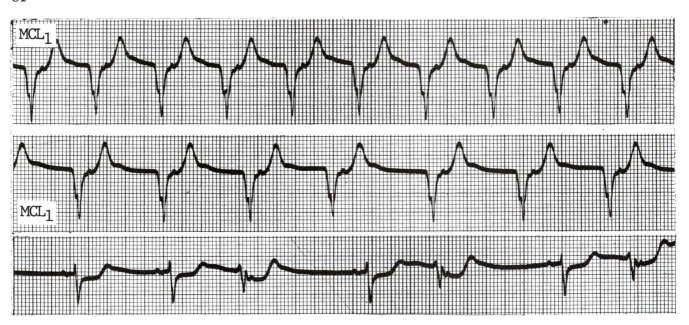

82

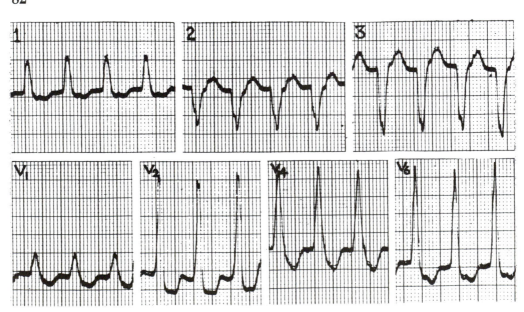

80

Diagnosis. **Sinus rhythm with intra-atrial block, first-degree A-V block** (P-R = 0.30 sec), and **ventricular trigeminy** (from a patient with digitalis intoxication).

Special Point. Intraatrial block can be diagnosed when the P wave measures 0.12 sec or more and is notched with two peaks more than 0.04 sec apart. Here, the P wave measures 0.14 sec and the peaks are 0.07 sec apart.

81

Diagnosis. Top strip: **AIVR** from the right ventricle (rate 88/min) with **1:1 retrograde conduction**. Middle strip: the same AIVR at a slower rate (about 64/min) and with some irregularity. Bottom strip: **sinus bradycardia** with **ventricular bigeminy**. (The ST-T pattern is due to the underlying acute inferior infarction.)

Special Point. Retrograde conduction to the atria is common in any ectopic ventricular rhythm. Note that idioventricular rhythms are not necessarily regular.

82

Diagnosis. **Left ventricular tachycardia** (rate 145/min) with **1:1 retrograde conduction.**

Special Points. This is the "concordant positivity" pattern (ventricular complexes positive across precordium from V_1 to V_6) that, provided you can exclude Wolff-Parkinson-White conduction, is virtually diagnostic of left ventricular ectopy. The marked left axis deviation also favors ventricular ectopy.

Retrograde P waves are well seen immediately after the QRS complexes in leads 1, 2, 3, and V_6. Retrograde conduction to the atria develops in about half of all ventricular tachycardias.[a,b]

[a] Kistin, A. D.: Retrograde conduction to the atria in ventricular tachycardia. Circulation *24*:236, 1961.
[b] Wellens, H. J. J., Bär, F. W., and Lie, K. I.: The value of the electrocardiogram in the differential diagnosis of a tachycardia with a widened QRS complex. Am. J. Med. *64*:27, 1978.

83

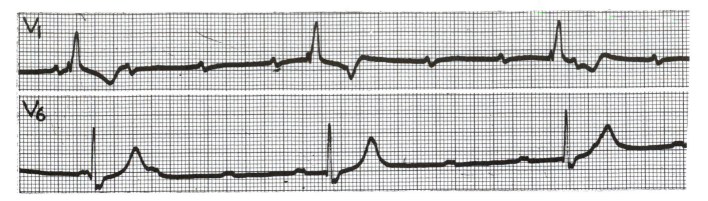

84

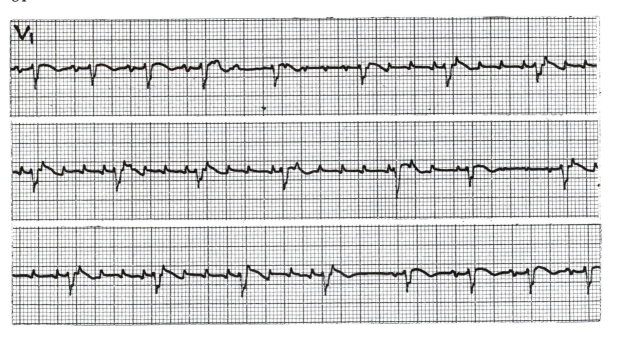

83

Diagnosis. **Sinus rhythm (rate 76/min) with complete A-V block** and **junctional escape** (rate 24/min) with **RBBB.**

Special Point. Although one cannot be absolutely sure of the junctional origin of the escape rhythm, the rsR´ pattern in V_1 and qRs in V_6 are so typical of RBBB that a supraventricular escape mechanism is far more likely than ventricular ectopy.

84

Diagnosis. **Sinus rhythm interrupted by a paroxysm of multifocal atrial tachycardia** with varying **A-V block.**

Special Point. Note that both the sinus P waves (beginning and end of strip) and the ectopic P´ waves are diphasic, but the sinus P waves are positive and then negative, the ectopic P waves are negative and then positive. This is the usual pattern of diphasic P waves in a right chest lead, such as V_1 or MCL_1.

85

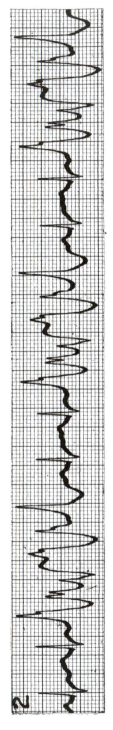

86

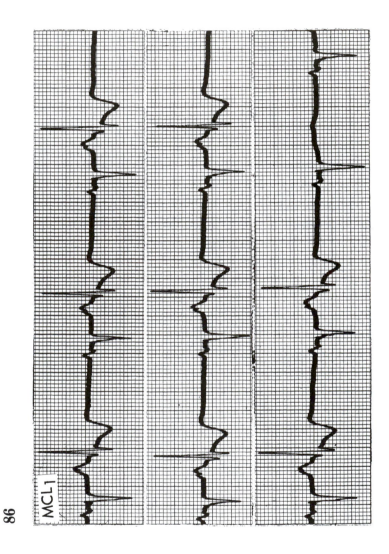

MCL1

85

Diagnosis. Sinus tachycardia with paroxysms of multiform, or polymorphous, **ventricular tachycardia.**

Special Point. This is from the same 32-year-old nurse as in Figure 6, who had no other evidence of heart disease. Note the remarkable similarity in the sequence of shapes in each paroxysm.

86

Diagnosis. Sinus bradycardia with **atrial bigeminy** with **aberrant ventricular conduction.**

Special Point. The morphology of the aberrant beats is interesting because it is not typical of either bundle-branch block. This may represent the unusual pattern of aberration described by Kulbertus,[a] now sometimes referred to as Kulbertus block.

[a] Kulbertus, H. E., deLaval-Rutten, F., and Custers, P.: Vectorcardiographic study of aberrant conduction. Anterior displacement of QRS: another form of intraventricular block. Br. Heart J. 38:549, 1976.

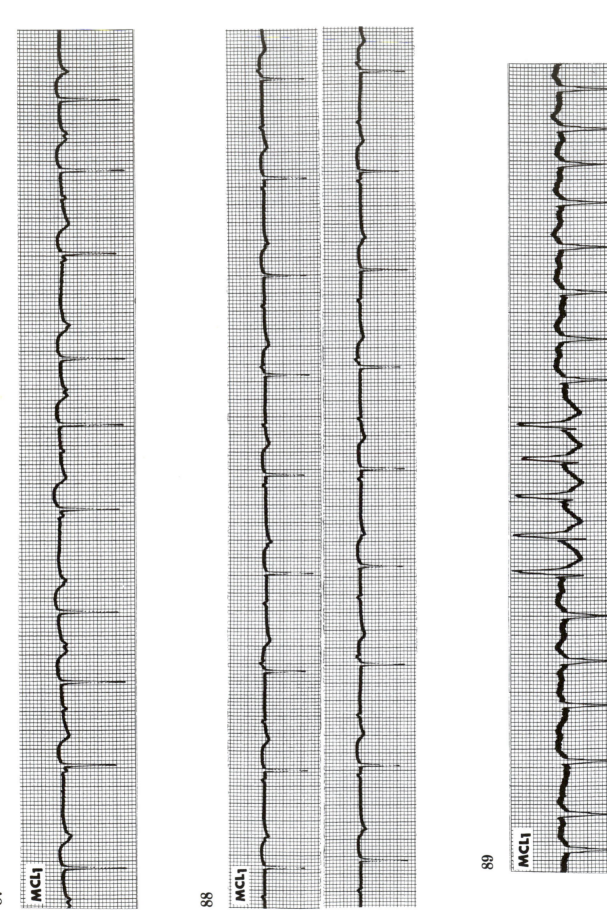

87

MCL₁

88

MCL₁

89

MCL₁

87

Diagnosis. Sinus rhythm at a rate of 90/min with A-V Wenckebach periods; junctional escape beats.

Special Point. The first ventricular complex in each trio ends a P-R interval much too short for conduction, especially in someone with Type I A-V block. Thus, in this case, the first QRS complex in each trio is clearly a junctional escape beat.

88

Diagnosis. (From the same patient as in Figure 87.) Some degree of Type I A-V block, combined with an atrial rate of 88/min and a junctional rate of 53/min, producing **complete A-V dissociation.**

Special Points. (1) The ventricular rate is too rapid to justify the label complete A-V block.

(2) The changed conduction pattern does not alter the *type* of block, which is still presumably A-V nodal or Type I. (3) Because there is no significant shortening of any of the *ventricular* cycles, one concludes that there is no A-V conduction.

89

Diagnosis. Atrial fibrillation with rapid ventricular response at about 130/min; a 5-beat run of **RBBB aberration.**

Special Point. The aberration is identified by the classic rSR´ of RBBB.

90

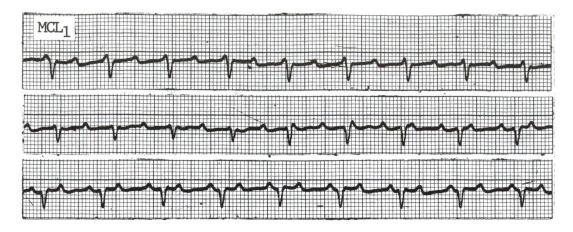

91

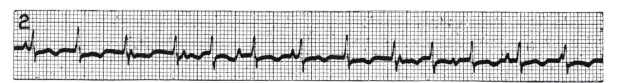

92

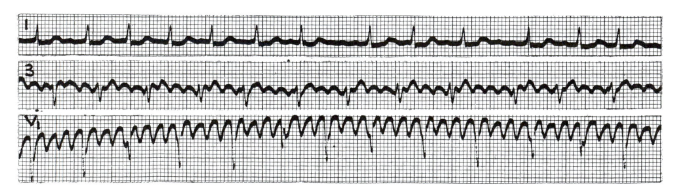

93

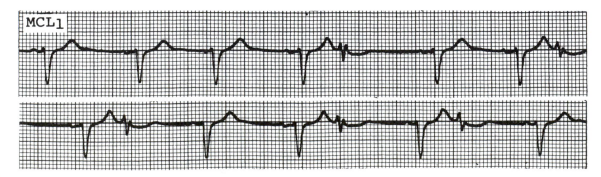

90

Diagnosis. **Atrial tachycardia** (rate 192/min) with **2:1 A-V conduction** and with progressively lengthening P′-R intervals. An equally plausible interpretation is complete dissociation between the two rhythms—atrial tachycardia and accelerated junctional (rate 96/min)—thanks to the **A-V block.**

Special Point. The top strip illustrates the "Bix Rule": whenever a P wave during a tachycardia is halfway between the QRS complexes, always suspect a P wave buried within the QRS complexes. This is an important caveat because, if there *is* 2:1 conduction and the atria are beating twice as fast as suspected, potential for a marked increase in the ventricular rate always exists, especially if the atria slow somewhat. Therapeutically, it is worthwhile to know of this danger.

91

Diagnosis. **Double tachycardia**—atrial (questionable sinus) at a rate of 106/min, junctional at a rate of 120/min—with frequent **ventricular captures.**

Special Point. The captures are recognized by shortening of the *ventricular* cycle: 5th, 6th, 10th, and 11th beats are captured.

92

Diagnosis. **Atrial flutter** (rate 415/min) with varying (mostly 4:1) conduction.

Special Point. This is an unusually rapid rate for atrial flutter; most have a rate between 250 and 320/min.

93

Diagnosis. **Sinus rhythm with frequent APBs** conducted with incomplete **RBBB aberration.**

Special Point. The T waves of the sinus beat immediately before the aberrant complexes appear taller and more pointed because of the superimposed premature P′ waves.

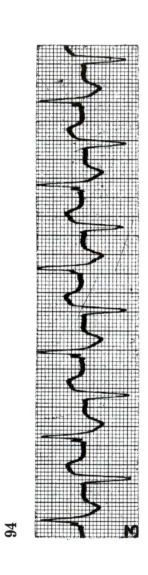

94

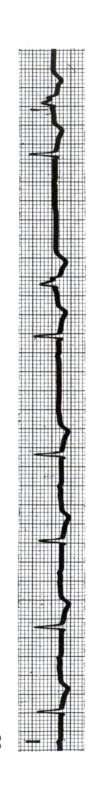

95

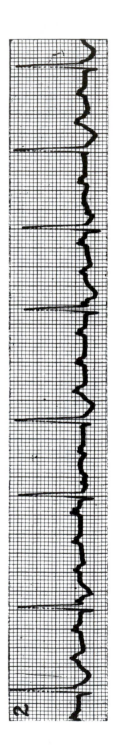

96

94

Diagnosis. Bidirectional tachycardia.

Special Point. The mechanism of this tachycardia may be junctional with RBBB and alternating anterior and posterior hemiblock or it may be ectopic ventricular with alternating pathways of ventricular activation (compare Figure 55).

95

Diagnosis. Sinus rhythm with first-degree A-V block (P-R = 0.34 sec); after a lengthened sinus cycle, **ventricular bigeminy** begins.

Special Point. This again illustrates the rule of bigeminy in action: lengthening of the ventricular cycle tends to precipitate a ventricular extrasystole, and the longer (postextrasystolic) cycle that results precipitates another. Hence, ventricular bigeminy tends to be self-perpetuating (compare Figures 64 and 68).

96

Diagnosis. Atrial tachycardia with varying **A-V block.** This arrhythmia was produced by digitalis intoxication and is often glibly referred to as "PAT with block." The P waves of the atrial tachycardia caused by digitalis intoxication are usually normally directed but smaller than average and somewhat irregular.

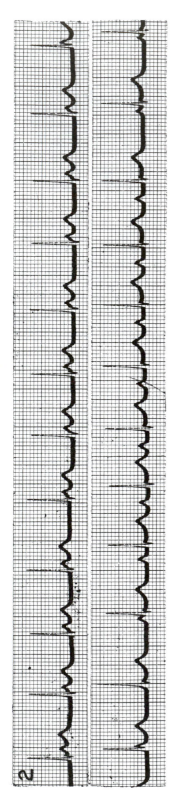

97

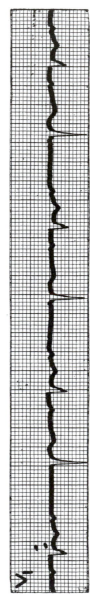

96

97

Diagnosis. Slightly irregular accelerated idiojunctional rhythm (rate 88/min) dissociated from the sinus rhythm of about the same rate (**isorhythmic A-V dissociation**). In the second strip, the sinus rhythm accelerates and assumes control of the ventricles with a slightly prolonged P-R interval (**first-degree A-V block**). At the end of the second strip, the sinus rhythm again slows, the junctional rhythm escapes, and dissociation recurs.

Treatment. Therapy depends on the cause of the accelerated junctional rhythm. The dysrhythmia itself requires no therapy unless the loss of atrial kick causes hemodynamic embarrassment.

98

Diagnosis. Sinus tachycardia (rate 106/min) with **Type I A-V block** manifesting itself as **escape-capture bigeminy;** enhanced junctional automaticity (potential escape rate of 62/min).

Special Point. This tracing is from an elderly man with an acute inferior infarction. When the sinus rhythm is accelerated, escape-capture bigeminy is a fairly common manifestation of Type I block, complicating acute inferior infarction, and accelerated junctional rhythms are quite common in this same context (see also Figure 104).

Treatment. None is usually required because (1) the ventricular rate (70/min) is adequate, (2) Type I A-V block in this context is always transient and has a good prognosis, and (3) accelerated junctional pacemakers are usually reliable.

99

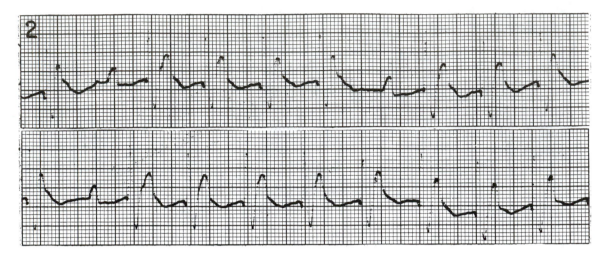

100

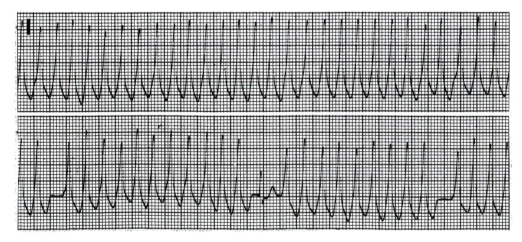

99

Diagnosis. Sinus tachycardia (rate 104/min) with **Type I A-V block** and **5:4 Wenckebach** periods; in the bottom strip a longer period begins.

Special Points. Most of the unusually large P waves look as though they were part of a much widened QRS complex. Note that although the P-R intervals are rather long, the successive increments are small (see laddergram).

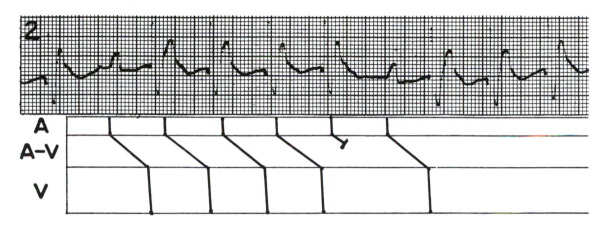

100

Diagnosis. Atrial fibrillation with conduction down an accessory pathway: bundle of Kent. (Tracing from a 19-year-old female with **Wolff-Parkinson-White syndrome**.)

Special Point. This sort of tracing has been misdiagnosed and published as ventricular tachycardia countless times. The diagnosis cannot be confirmed from the tracing alone, but it is so typical of atrial fibrillation with ventricular preexcitation that it is unlikely to be anything else. Clues to the correct diagnosis include cycles representing a rate approximating 300/min, with cycles elsewhere that are more than twice as long as the shortest cycles. This disparity represents a degree of irregularity unlikely to be seen in ventricular tachycardia.

101

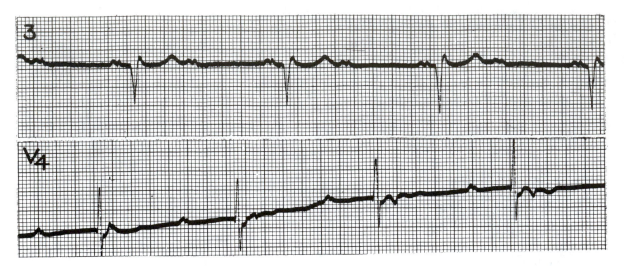

102

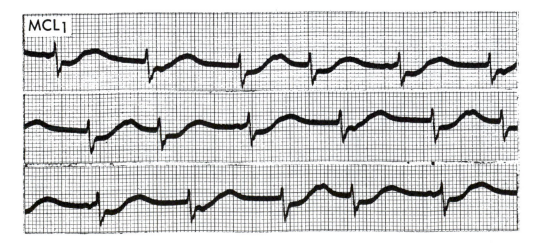

101

Diagnosis. **Sinus rhythm with intra-atrial block, complete A-V block, idiojunctional rhythm** (rate 38–43/min), and **RBBB; retrograde conduction** to atria with **atrial fusion.**

Special Points. P waves measure 0.12 sec in duration and have peaks more than 0.04 sec apart. This qualifies as intraatrial block.

At first inspection of lead 3, 2 : 1 block might be suspected, but careful measurement shows that the P-R intervals are gradually shrinking (the first is 0.22 sec and the last is 0.17 sec). Moreover, in lead V_4, the P-R intervals are quite different but show similar progressive decrease (from 0.67 to 0.45 sec); clearly, the P waves and QRS complexes are dissociated.

The terminal wide r wave in lead 3 and S in V_4 are so characteristic of RBBB that one suspects the site of the complete A-V block to be above the bifurcation of the A-V bundle.

Finally, although anterograde block is presumably complete, retrograde conduction is clearly facile, as manifested after the last two beats in V_4. The P wave immediately after the second QRS in lead V_4 occupies a position at which both sinus P and retrograde P could be expected. However, it has the shape of neither and therefore clearly represents atrial fusion (see laddergram).

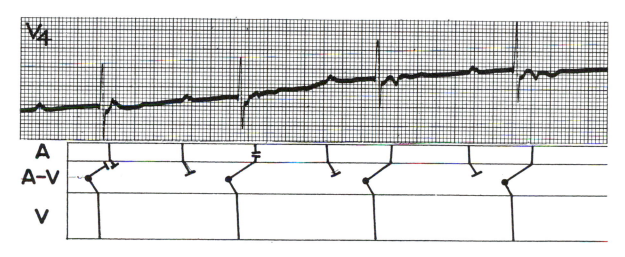

102

Diagnosis. **Sinus bradycardia** (rate 50/min) with an **accelerated junctional rhythm** (rate 62/min) produces **A-V dissociation** with frequent **ventricular captures;** mild **A-V block.** (From a patient with combined digitalis and quinidine effects; note the ST-T-U contour.)

Special Point. The capture beats (fourth beat in the top strip, second and last beats in the second strip, and fourth beat in the bottom strip) are readily recognized *because they end shorter cycles* than the independent junctional cycles. Judging by the prolonged P-R intervals of the captured beats, there is some A-V block, but this does not contribute to the dissociation.

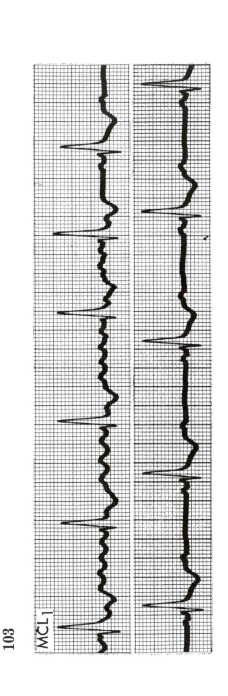

103

MCL₁

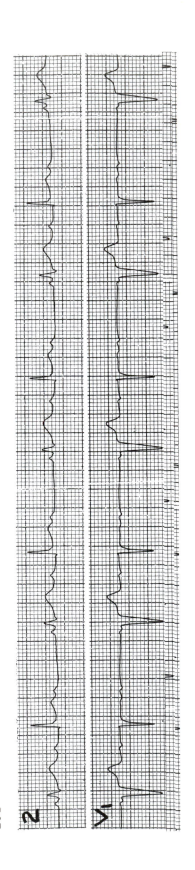

104

2

V₁

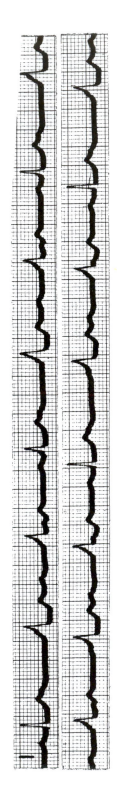

105

103

Diagnosis. Atrial flutter-fibrillation giving place to sinus rhythm with 2 : 1 **Type II A-V block; RBBB.**

Special Point. During the 2 : 1 conduction, the combination of normal P-R interval with bundle-branch block strongly suggests, but does not prove, that the block is Type II, that is, infranodal.

104

Diagnosis. Sinus rhythm (rate 98/min) with Type I A-V block and **ventricular escape,** producing one form of **escape-capture bigeminy.**

Special Points. The conducted beats have a prolonged P-R interval and no bundle-branch block, identifying the block almost certainly as Type I. After each dropped beat, the ventricle escapes before the next atrial impulse can be conducted, resulting in this rather common form of escape-capture bigeminy (compare Figure 86).

105

Diagnosis. Sinus tachycardia (rate 102/min) with **intraatrial block** and some degree of **Type I A-V block,** permitting an **accelerated idioventricular rhythm** (rate 62/min) to escape for from two to four consecutive beats. In the upper strip, the fourth and seventh beats are **fusion beats.**

106

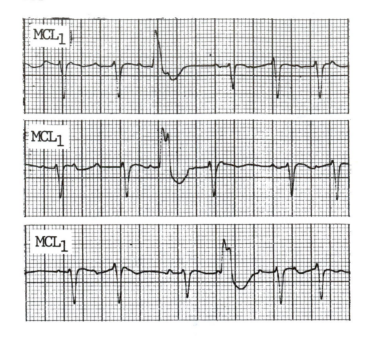

107

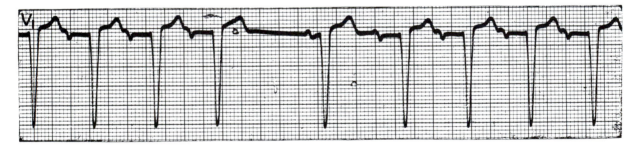

106

Diagnosis. **Sinus tachycardia** with **left VPBs,** including one **fusion beat; numerous APBs.**

Special Point. Looking at the top strip alone, one might immediately diagnose the third beat as an APB with ventricular aberration. However, the fact that the QRS peaks early with slurring on the downstroke raises the suspicion of ectopy. Further, when one scans the lower strips in which the anomalous ventricular complexes have obviously taller left rabbit ears, identical coupling intervals, and P-R intervals impossibly short for A-V conduction, it becomes obvious that the third beat in the top strip is much more likely a fusion beat between an APB and a VPB.

107

Diagnosis. **Sinus rhythm (rate 90/min) with first-degree A-V block,** interrupted by a nonconducted **APB** followed by **junctional escape.** After the escape beat, sinus rhythm with first-degree A-V block resumes.

Special Points. The premature P′ wave is recognized by the change in the fourth ST-T: all others are concave upward, whereas the fourth ST-T has lost that concavity.

The returning beat is almost certainly escape rather than conducted; although its P-R interval (0.14 sec) is certainly compatible with conduction, it is unlikely that a heart with first-degree block and a P-R interval of 0.28 sec would conduct with a so much shorter interval, even after such a long R-P interval.

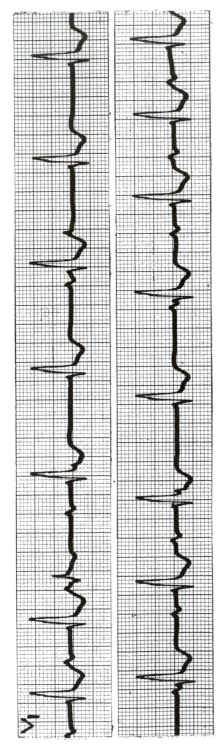

108

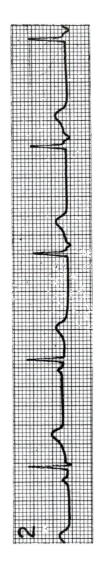

109

108

Diagnosis. **Sinus rhythm at a rate of 75/min with Type I A-V block** and **RBBB; junctional escape** rhythm at 56/min; one **VPB** and three nonconducted **APBs.**

Special Points. The first two beats are conducted with prolonged P-R intervals (about 0.40 sec). The third beat is a VPB and is probably followed by a conducted beat and then a nonconducted APB; the pause after this ends with junctional escape, and there is then a run of five es-

cape beats (idiojunctional rhythm). Conduction resumes with the second and third beats in the bottom strip, *recognized by the fact that these beats end cycles shorter than the escape cycles.* Two more junctional escapes follow and then the strip ends with three more conducted sinus beats. These last three beats prove that the A-V block is of the Type I class because they show a clear re-ciprocal relationship between their R-P and P-R intervals.

109

Diagnosis. **Shifting** (or wandering) pace-maker, with one dissociated and one **atrial fu-sion beat** (see laddergram).

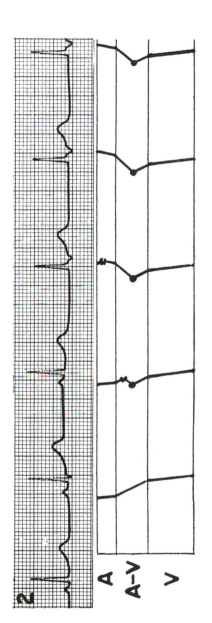

110

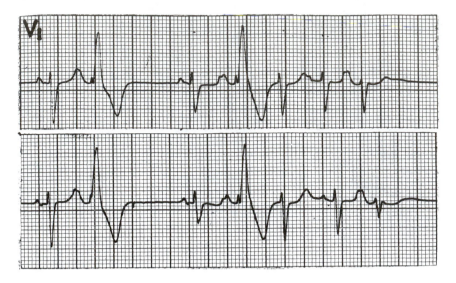

111

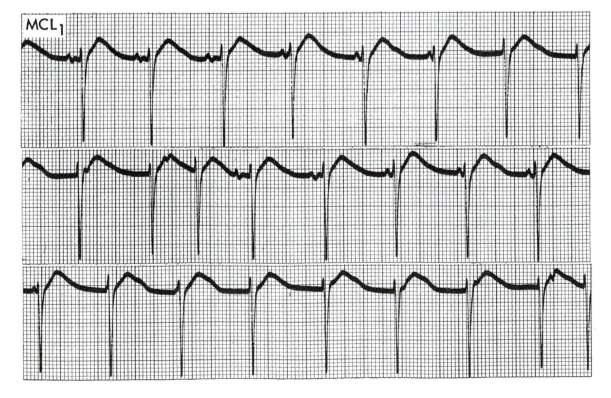

110

Diagnosis. **Sinus rhythm interrupted by APBs,** both singly and in runs of four, **atrial tachycardia;** the isolated APBs and the first in each salvo of four are conducted with **RBBB aberration.**

Special Point. Note that the last beat in the bottom strip ends a shorter cycle than the preceding beats and shows the earliest signs of RBBB aberration, namely, shrinkage of the S wave and a rudimentary r´.

111

Diagnosis. **Accelerated junctional rhythm** at a rate of 80/min usurping control from a normal sinus rhythm (rate 76/min) and producing **A-V dissociation.** The third and fourth beats in the second strip and the last beat in the bottom strip are **ventricular captures.**

Special Points. Note the prolonged P-R intervals in two of the capture beats and the reciprocal R-P/P-R relationship in the two capture beats in the middle strip.

Treatment. There is no specific treatment for accelerated junctional rhythm, unless it is attributable to some removable cause, such as digitalis intoxication. In this case it was secondary to an acute inferior infarction. If the loss of atrial kick proves to be hemodynamically embarrassing, a cautious attempt may be made with atropine to increase the sinus rate sufficiently to recapture the ventricles.

112

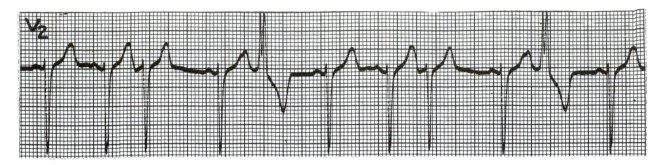

113

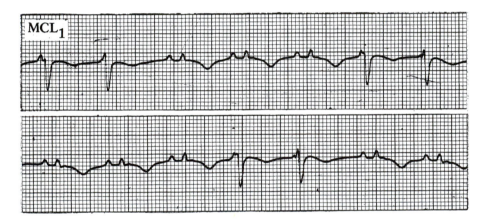

114

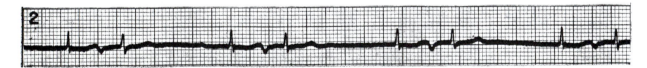

112

Diagnosis. **The sinus rhythm is interrupted by frequent APBs, two of which are conducted with RBBB aberration.**

Special Point. Why are the second and fourth APBs conducted aberrantly, whereas the others are not? Unlike the situation in Figure 35, the aberrant complexes do not end shorter cycles and therefore greater prematurity is not the explanation. The answer lies in the preceding cycle. The normally conducted APB suppresses the sinus node (overdrive suppression) and so lengthens the following cycle; this cycle, in turn, lengthens the ensuing refractory period of the ventricular conduction system and favors the development of aberration.

113

Diagnosis. **After each trio of sinus beats (rate 88/min), a pair of ectopic ventricular beats at an accelerated rate (95/min) usurps control.**

Special Point. This suggests the potential for an accelerated idioventricular rhythm, but for some reason the usurping ventricular rhythm always retires after two beats.

114

Diagnosis. Junctional rhythm with reciprocal bigeminy (see laddergram).

Special Point. This rhythm should make one think of digitalis intoxication.

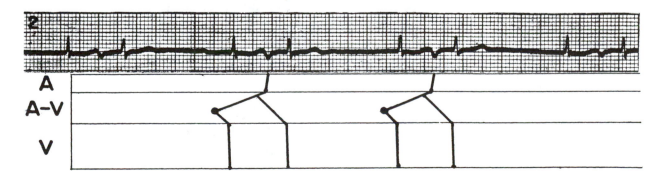

115

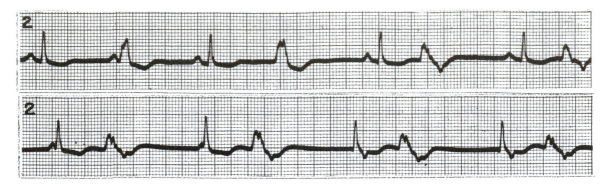

116

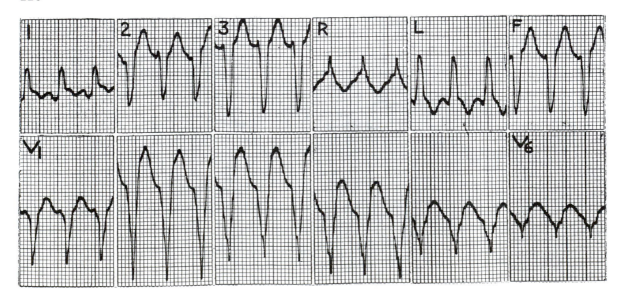

115

Diagnosis. **Top strip: sinus rhythm with VPBs** with varying "coupling" intervals. The interectopic intervals, however, do not measure convincingly for parasystole. The last two ectopic beats are conducted retrogradely to the atria with R-P intervals of 0.24 sec. Bottom strip: junctional rhythm with ventricular bigeminy. The first two junctional beats are dissociated from the sinus rhythm; the last two manifest retrograde conduction to the atria with R-P intervals of 0.12 sec. All VPBs show retrograde conduction to the atria with R-P intervals of 0.24 sec.

Special Point. Note that in the same heart, retrograde conduction differs in junctional and ventricular ectopic beats. This is because in ventricular beats the R-P interval is a direct measurement of retrograde conduction, whereas in junctional beats the R-P represents the difference between anterograde and retrograde conduction (see diagram). Key: a = junctional beat; b = ectopic ventricular beat; c = a and b superimposed.

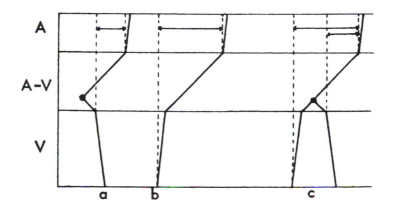

116

Diagnosis. **Right ventricular tachycardia** (rate 168/min).

Special Points. Features identifying this tachycardia are the marked left axis deviation (−90°), concordant negativity in the V leads, and QRS duration of more than 0.14 sec.

117

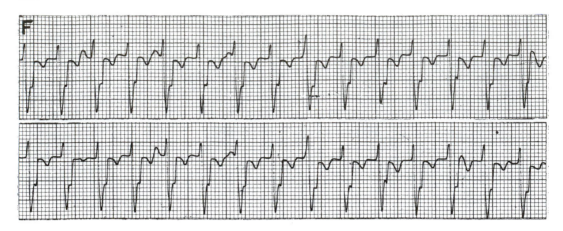

118

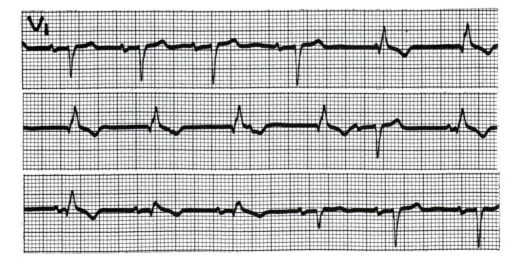

117

Diagnosis. Ventricular tachycardia (rate 160/min).

Special Points. From this single lead, the strongest point favoring ventricular tachycardia is the independent P waves (arrows). This happens to be the form of ventricular tachycardia that imitates RBBB plus left anterior hemiblock (see other reproduced leads), usually found in otherwise healthy, young people with no other evidence of heart disease.

Treatment. This is the one form of ventricular tachycardia that frequently responds to verapamil.[a]

[a] Lin, F.-C., Finley, C. D., Rahimtoola, S. H., and Wu, D.: Idiopathic paroxysmal ventricular tachycardia with a QRS pattern of right bundle branch block and left axis deviation: a unique clinical entity with specific properties. Am. J. Cardiol. *52*:95, 1983.

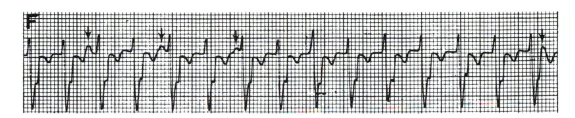

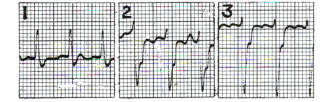

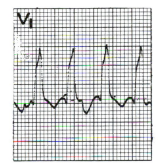

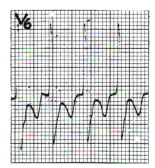

118

Diagnosis. **Sinus arrhythmia,** the bradycrotic phase of which enables an **accelerated idioventricular rhythm** to take over. The fifth beat in the middle strip is a **ventricular capture,** and the second through fourth beats in the bottom strip are **fusion beats.**

Special Point. Remember that AIVR always takes over either because the sinus rhythm slows (A-V dissociation by default) or the AIVR accelerates (A-V dissociation by usurpation).

119

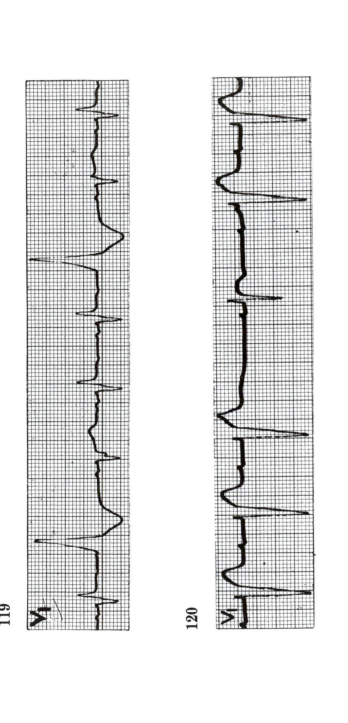

120

121

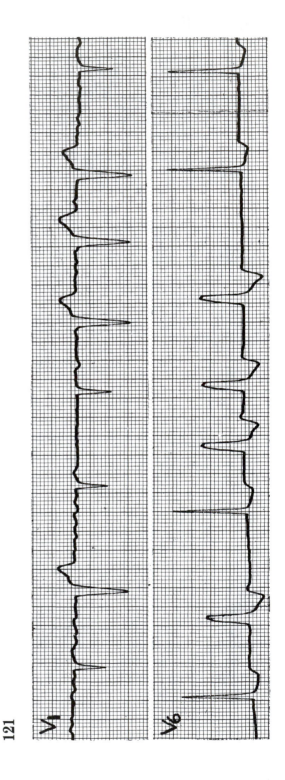

119

Diagnosis. Sinus rhythm with rate-dependent RBBB; left **VPBs.**

Special Point. One recognizes that the RBBB is rate dependent by the improved intraventricular conduction in the beats ending the longer cycles after each VPB; both of these postectopic beats manifest lesser degrees of RBBB.

Note that the earliest indication of RBBB in lead V_1 is a slurring or notching on the upstroke of the S wave, as in the beat after the first VPB. A slightly more advanced stage of RBBB produces a tiny r′, as in the beat after the second VPB.

In other cases, the earliest manifestation of RBBB is a shrinkage of the S wave (see Figures 146, 161 and 209).

120

Diagnosis. Sinus rhythm with first-degree A-V block (P-R = 0.31 sec) **with rate-dependent LBBB; nonconducted APB.**

Special Point. As in Figure 119, the BBB is recognized as rate dependent from the improved conduction in the beat ending the long cycle occasioned by the nonconducted APB.

The concomitant shortening of the P-R interval in the postectopic beat suggests that the A-V block is also rate related; however, the apparent P-R shortening might be because the postectopic beat is an escape beat.

121

Diagnosis. Atrial fibrillation with controlled ventricular response and **rate-dependent LBBB.**

Special Point. Note that all cycles of 0.92 sec or shorter end with LBBB, whereas all cycles of 1.00 sec or longer end with more normally conducted beats. (The ST-T configuration of these beats suggests digitalis effect superimposed on left ventricular hypertrophy.)

122

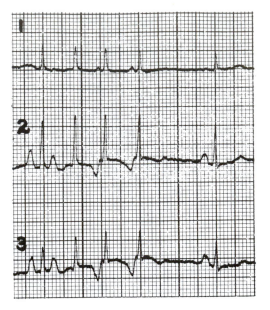

123

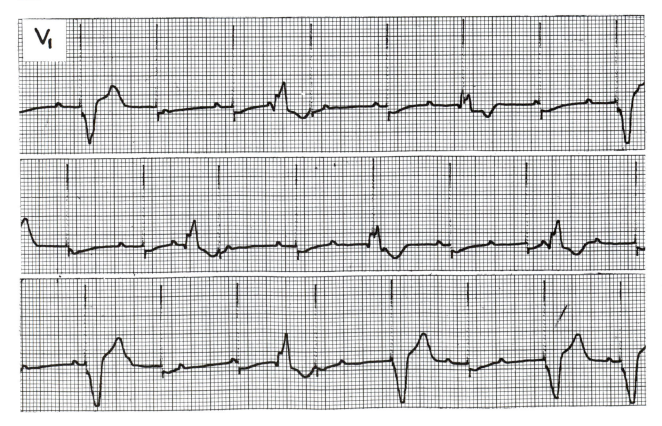

122

Diagnosis. Although we do not know what preceded it, the first beat is probably an APB, and the second beat is certainly one with a prolonged P-R interval. This delayed conduction favors reentry and a **reciprocating mechanism** is set up, probably using an accessory pathway in the posterior septum for the retrograde path, but it lasts for only two cycles. The final beat is presumably a sinus beat.

Retrograde P waves, inverted in leads 2, 3, and aVF, are often, as in this case, upright in lead 1.

123

Diagnosis. Complete A-V block with **left idioventricular rhythm** at a rate of 30/min; intermittently ineffective demand **right ventricular pacemaker.** The third ventricular complex in the top strip and the second in the middle strip represent **fusion** between idioventricular and paced impulses. The only appropriately sensed beat is the last beat in the middle strip.

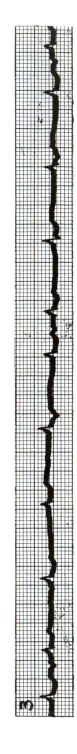

124

3

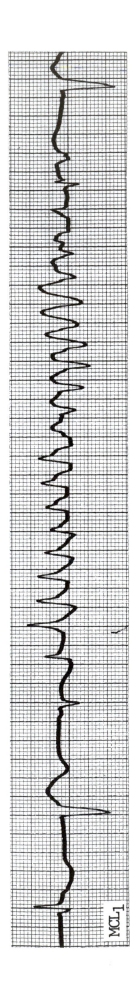

125

MCL_1

124

Diagnosis. **Junctional rhythm** with **reciprocal beating** (see laddergram).

Special Point. Whenever apparently retrograde P waves marching through supraventricular QRS complexes and then an early beat are seen, there are always two possibilities: junctional rhythm with progressive delay in retrograde conduction and reciprocal beats or A–V dissociation between a higher and a lower junctional rhythm with ventricular captures by the upper pacemaker. Simply measuring the P-P intervals usually differentiates them. If two junctional pacemakers are dissociated, the P-P intervals are usually constant because junctional pacemakers are almost always regular (see Figure 181). However, if the location of the P waves is dependent on varying retrograde conduction, the P-P intervals, as in this case, usually vary but bear a recurring relationship to the QRS complexes.

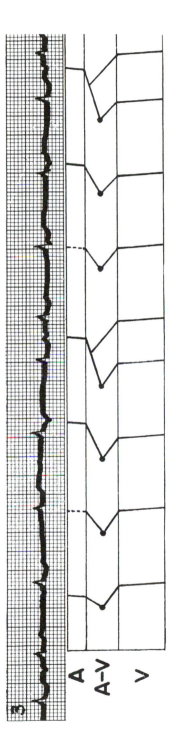

A
A–V
V

125

Diagnosis. **After two bifocal ventricular ectopic beats** at a slow rate, a sinus beat is followed by a **VPB**, interrupting its T wave and precipitating a paroxysm of **torsades de pointes.**

Special Points. Note that the direction of the QRS complex during the paroxysm swings from positive to negative and that there are many differently shaped QRS complexes (polymorphous ventricular tachycardia). Note also that the Q-T interval of the sinus beat is obviously prolonged.

126

MCL₁

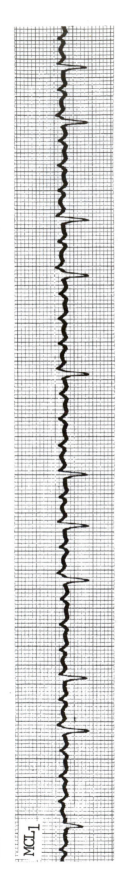

127

MCL₁

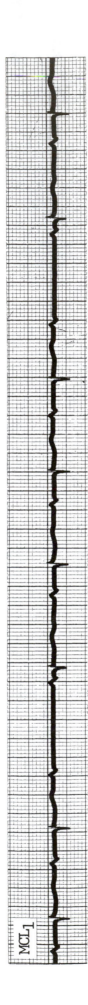

126

Diagnosis. Atrial tachycardia (rate 220/min) with 2:1 and 4:1 A-V conduction.

Special Points. Note that within each pair or trio of ventricular beats there is a progressive lengthening of the A-V conduction (P′-R) interval. This is because at a lower level in the junction, below the constant 2:1 filter, Wenckebach conduction is occurring (see laddergram). Notice also that the P′ wave immediately preceding the QRS complex does not represent the atrial impulse

that is conducted—it is usually the one before that. This is because of the concealed conduction into the junction. Constant bombardment of the A-V node by so many atrial impulses keeps the junction partially refractory. The conducted F-R intervals in atrial flutter are usually thought to be between 0.26 and 0.46 sec.[a]

---

[a] Besoain-Santander, M, Pick, A., and Langendorf, R.: A-V conduction in auricular flutter. Circulation 2:604, 1950.

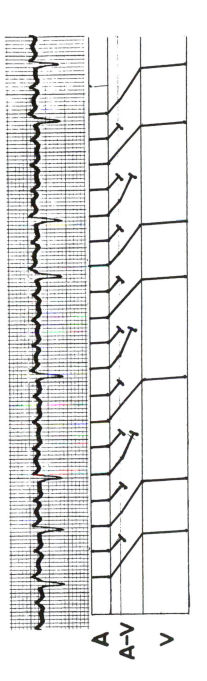

A

A–V

V

127

Diagnosis. Sinus rhythm (rate 64/min) with A-V Wenckebach periods.

Special Point. Note that in the complete Wenckebach period shown, consecutive P-R intervals are 17, 33, 37, and 39—a classic progression. But in most Wenckebach periods, even the first

P-R is longer than normal, and the possibility therefore arises that in this case the first QRS complex may represent junctional escape rather than A-V conduction. Moreover, the jump from 17 to 33 is unusually large for even the maximal P-R increment.

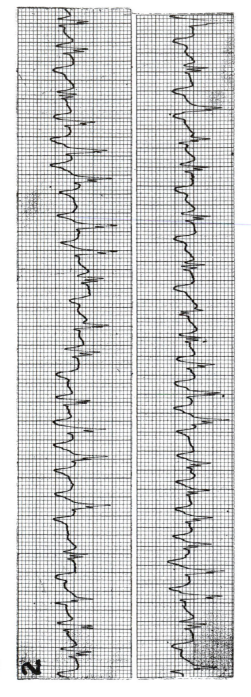

128

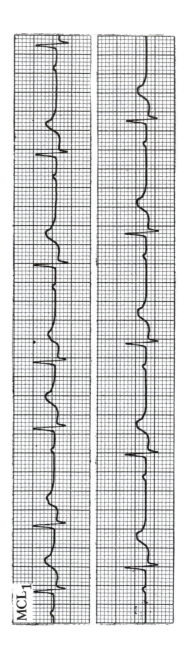

129

128

Diagnosis. Atrial tachycardia (rate 226/min) with repeated **Wenckebach periods.** Note that the negative QRS in lead 2 indicates an abnormal axis, probably leftward.

Special Points. The apparent change in the contour of the QRS complex from beat to beat is entirely due to its changing relationship to the sizable P wave.

The presence of even this mild failure of A-V conduction establishes the tachycardia as ectopic atrial and excludes a reentrant mechanism.

129

Diagnosis. Sinus tachycardia (rate 102/min) with 3 : 2 and 2 : 1 **Type I A-V block.** (From a patient with acute inferoposterior myocardial infarction. Note the reciprocal changes—dominant R wave, ST segment depression, and upright T wave—of true posterior wall involvement.)

130

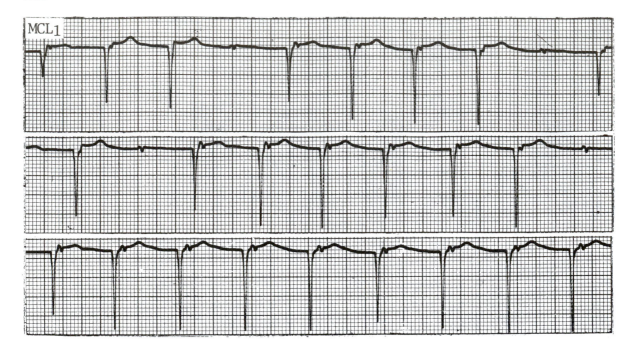

131

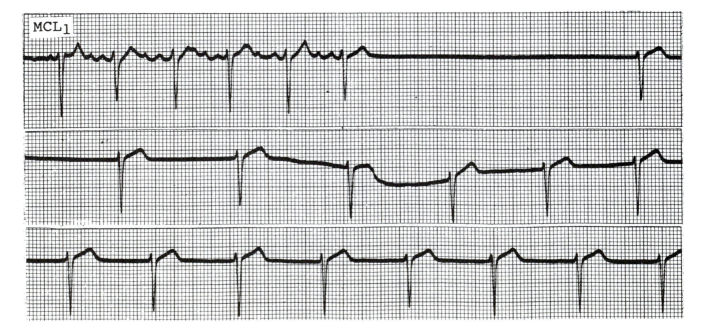

130

Diagnosis. **Sinus rhythm (rate 92/min) with Type I A-V block** in the form of 5 : 4, 3 : 2, and 7 : 6 **Wenckebach periods.**

Special Points. Note (1) the P-R intervals that are nearly as long as the R-R intervals, (2) the minimal P-R increments, and (3) the way the P-R interval settles down to a constant 0.60 sec in the bottom strip.

131

Diagnosis. **Sick sinus syndrome** manifested by **atrial fibrillation** and then complete absence of any atrial activity (**tachycardia-bradycardia syndrome**). After a 3-sec pause, the junction escapes and then warms up to an accelerated rate of 68/min.

Treatment. Unless the disturbance is secondary to an acute removable process, a permanent pacemaker is indicated, preferably in the AAI mode.

132

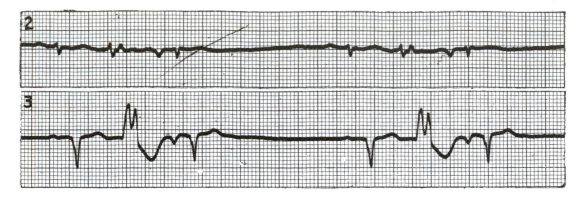

133

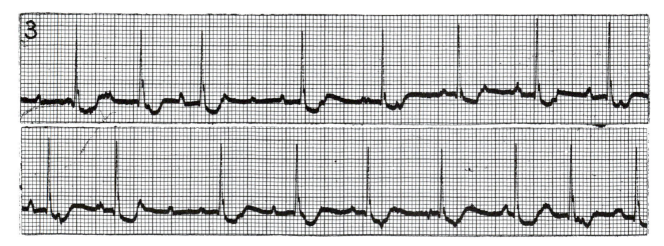

132

Diagnosis. **Sinus rhythm with ventricular extrasystoles** followed by retrograde conduction and **reciprocal beats,** in this context sometimes called "return extrasystoles" (see laddergram).

Special Point. Note the long R-P interval (0.50 sec) favoring the development of reentry. Compare also Figures 174 and 184. Because conducted P-R intervals can occasionally measure a full second or so, an R-P interval this long should not be a surprise.

133

Diagnosis. **Multifocal atrial tachycardia** with varying **A-V block** (due to digitalis intoxication).

Special Point. Note the sagging ST segments with relatively short Q-T intervals highly suggestive of digitalis effect.

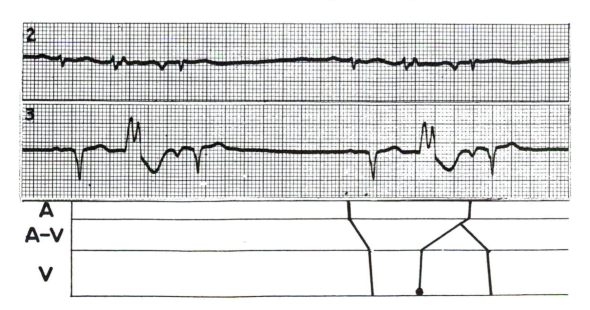

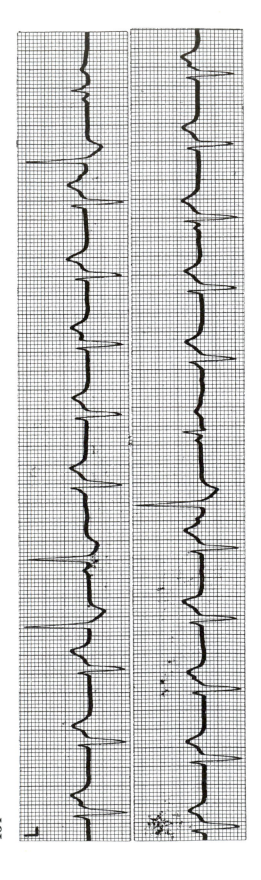

134

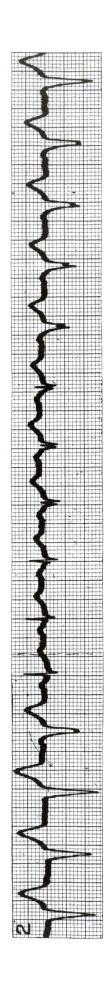

135

134

Diagnosis. **Accelerated idioventricular rhythm** (rate 80/min) producing **A-V dissociation** from a normal sinus rhythm that has a rate of 72/min. The upright complexes are **ventricular captures** (their pattern suggests left ventricular hypertrophy). The 5th and 12th beats in the top strip and the 7th in the bottom strip are **fusion beats** between sinus and idioventricular impulses.

135

Diagnosis. **Accelerated idioventricular rhythm** (rate 94/min) producing **A-V dissociation** from a sinus rhythm with a similar rate. In the middle of the strip, the sinus rhythm accelerates to produce a string of **fusion beats** and possibly some complete captures. The 5th, 6th, and 7th beats may be pure sinus beats or may be fusion beats; the 4th and 8th through 14th beats are undoubtedly fusion beats.

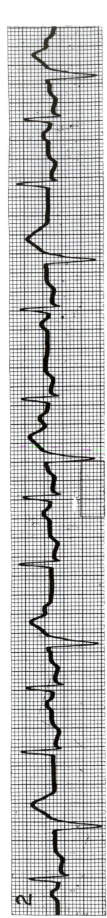

136

Diagnosis. **Sinus rhythm interrupted by interpolated VPBs** with **concealed retrograde conduction** lengthening the ensuing P-R intervals.

Special Point. Note that the R-P interval after each VPB determines the P-R interval, in the same way that the R-P and P-R intervals are reciprocally related in Type I A-V block. This is because the retrograde conduction sets up a refractory period, and the shorter the ensuing R-P interval, the earlier the attempt of the sinus impulse to penetrate that refractory period (see laddergram). Thus, the R-P:P-R ratios for the three VPBs diagrammed are 30:53, 40:48, and 44:22.

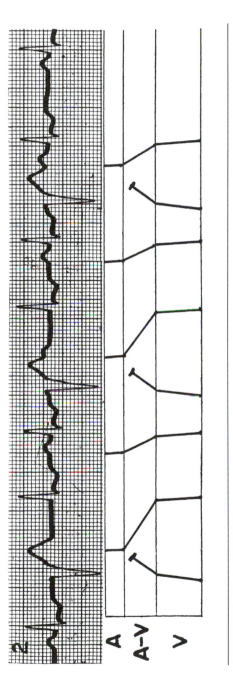

137

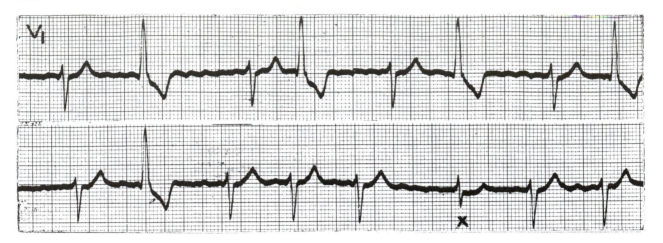

138

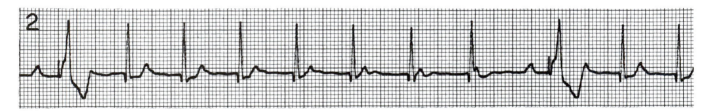

139

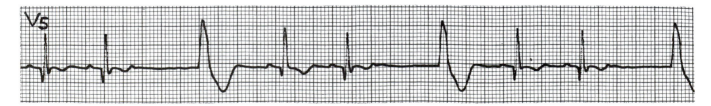

137

Diagnosis. **Atrial fibrillation** with controlled ventricular response; **left ventricular parasystole** (rate 36/min); one **fusion beat** (x).

Special Point. Note that the interectopic intervals in the top strip are all virtually identical, and in the bottom strip, the interval from the ectopic beat to the fusion beat is exactly double.

Treatment. Usually, parasystole is benign and requires no treatment, unless it is due to a removable cause such as digitalis intoxication.

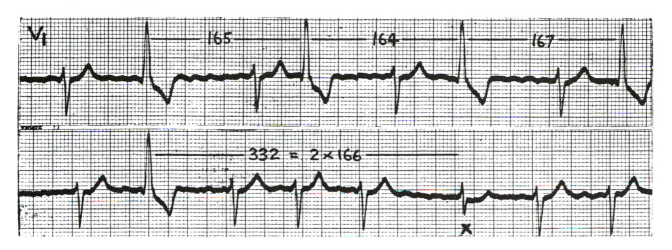

138

Diagnosis. Sinus rhythm (rate 100/min), with A-V Wenckebach period; demand pacemaker escapes after dropped beat.

Special Point. Between the two paced beats is an 8 : 7 Wenckebach period in which the P-R is almost as long as the R-R interval. (One or two A-V Wenckebach periods are illustrated later in which the P-R is actually longer than the R-R interval.)

Treatment. No further treatment is required; the only question is whether the pacemaker was really necessary.

139

Diagnosis. After each pair of sinus beats, a nonconducted APB is followed by a long enough cycle for **ventricular escape** to occur. But the ventricular focus is escaping at a rate of about 60/min, so there is the potential for an AIVR to develop at that rate.

140

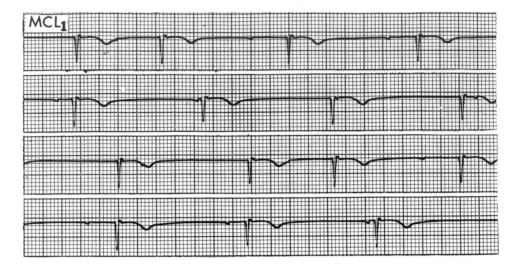

141

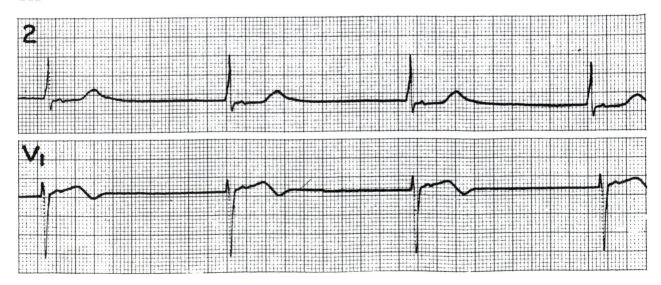

140

Diagnosis. Sinus bradycardia (rate 40/min) with resulting **junctional escape** (rate 44/min) and **A-V dissociation;** two **ventricular captures** with prolonged P-R intervals of 0.46–0.48 sec.

Special Point. Once again, it is the shortened ventricular cycle that alerts one to the fact that conduction (capture) has occurred (second beat in top strip and third beat in third strip).

141

Diagnosis. **Sick sinus syndrome** with **junctional escape** at a rate of 32/min with **retrograde conduction** to the atria.

Special Point. Although the *rhythm* is junctional, keep in mind that the primary *diag-*

nosis is a sick sinus. It is impossible to have a junction in control at this rate unless the sinus is ailing.

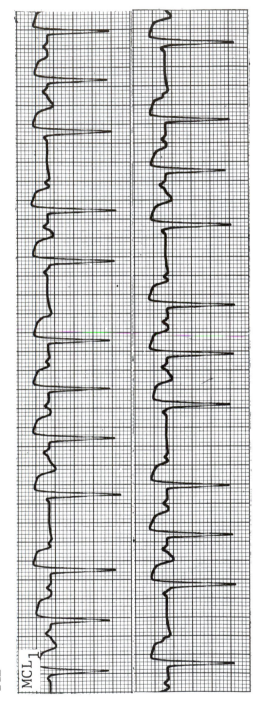

MCL₁

142

Diagnosis. Sinus tachycardia (rate 126/min) with 5:4, 4:3, and 3:2 **Wenckebach periods** (see laddergram).

Special Points. Besides the obvious lengthening of the P-R intervals and the recurring P to R relationships, all the "footprints" of the A-V Wenckebach period are in place: small groups of beats, progressive shortening of R-R intervals within the group, and the longest R-R intervals less than twice the shortest.

Many at first find it difficult to accept the fact that the conducted atrial impulse can be represented by a P wave situated in front of the previous QRS complex; in colloquial idiom, they find it difficult to understand how a P wave can be con-

ducted "over the top of" a QRS to the next QRS. But, of course, this lack of acceptance stems from the artifact of recording, side by side on two-dimensional paper, events that are happening at quite different levels in the heart. If the sinus node has a mandate to beat at 126 beats/min, it will beat at 126 beats/min: when it is time to deliver its next impulse, it does not matter whether the previous impulse has yet reached the ventricles, an event that is taking place in a region of the heart remote to the sinus node. With Type I A-V block and sinus or atrial tachycardia, it is not uncommon for the P-R interval to exceed the R-R interval and for this sort of "skip" conduction to result.

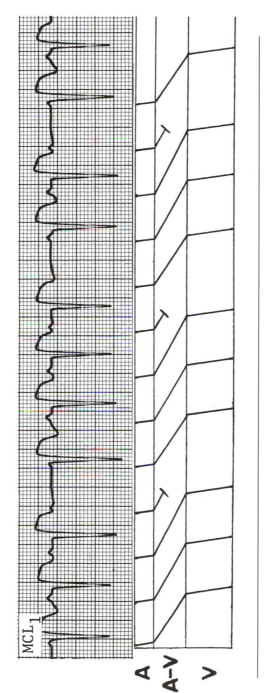

143

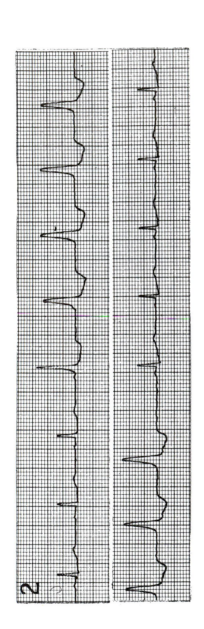

144

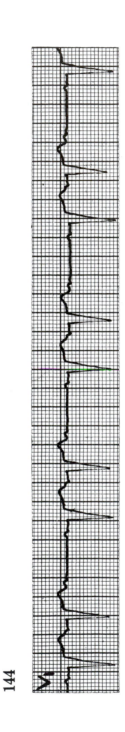

145

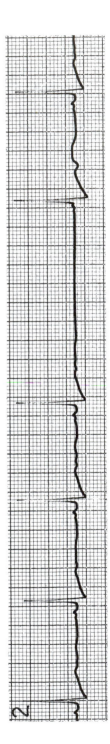

143

Diagnosis. After three sinus beats, an **AIVR** at 88/min takes over via one **fusion beat** (the fourth beat). In the bottom strip, the AIVR abruptly ceases, enabling the sinus rhythm to regain control.

Treatment. The great majority of AIVRs require no treatment; however, if the loss of atrial kick produces hemodynamic embarrassment, an attempt must be made to restore the normal A-V contraction sequence. Atropine, in a cautious dosage, may be tried to accelerate the sinus rhythm, or an attempt may be made to suppress the ectopic rhythm with an antiarrhythmic agent.

144

Diagnosis. Sinus tachycardia (rate 115/min) with 3:2 **Type II A-V block; LBBB.**

Treatment. As this is undoubtedly genuine Type II block, with its normal P-R interval, bun-dle-branch block, and unchanging P-R intervals when *consecutive* beats are conducted before the dropped beat, a pacemaker is certainly indicated.

145

Diagnosis. Sick sinus syndrome mani-fested as **Type II sinoatrial block.**

Special Point. By analogy with Type II A-V block, it is called Type II sinoatrial block when the longer cycle is a multiple of the shorter (see figure). If it were Type I block, the long cycle would be less than twice the shorter cycles.

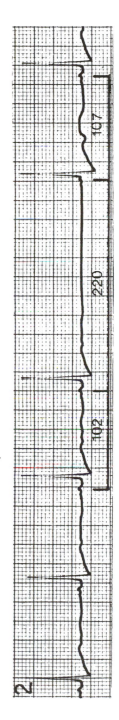

146

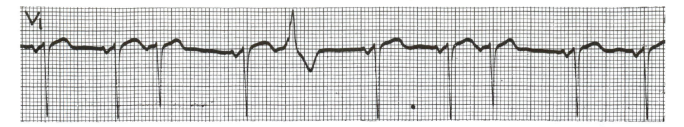

147

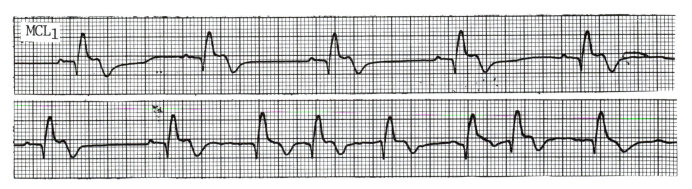

148

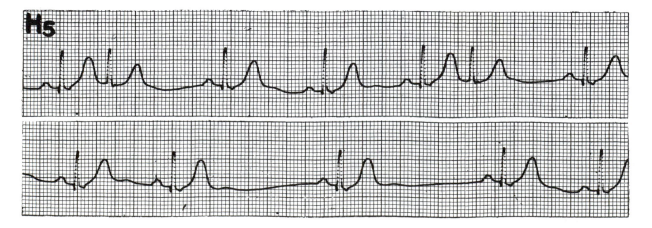

146

Diagnosis. Sinus rhythm interrupted by three **APBs**, the second showing **RBBB aberration**.

Special Point. Why is the second APB conducted with RBBB aberration, whereas the other two are not? (As a matter of fact, even they are beginning to show the first sign of aberration; there is actually a reduction in the depth of their S waves, often the earliest sign of RBBB.) The cycle preceding the first and third APBs is a pure sinus cycle, beginning and ending with a sinus beat, whereas the cycle preceding the frankly aberrant beat begins with an APB, which by overdrive suppression momentarily stuns the sinus node and thus lengthens the cycle. And because the refractory periods of all parts of the ventricular conduction system are proportional to the length of the preceding cycle, the likelihood for aberration is thus enhanced.

147

Diagnosis. **Top strip: sinus rhythm with RBBB** and **nonconducted atrial bigeminy.** Bottom strip: the second APB precipitates **atrial fibrillation.** (The Q wave, slightly elevated ST segment, and frankly inverted T waves proclaim the underlying anteroseptal myocardial infarction.)

Special Point. Nonconducted atrial bigeminy simulates sinus bradycardia and may invite overdiagnosis of a sick sinus syndrome. Therefore, whenever sinus bradycardia is suspected, always look carefully in the neighborhood of the T waves for lurking P′ waves.

148

Diagnosis. **APBs,** conducted in top strip and nonconducted in bottom strip.

Special Point. Nonconducted APBs, especially when P′ waves are undetected, simulate sinus pauses and may lead to an overdiagnosis of sick sinus syndrome.

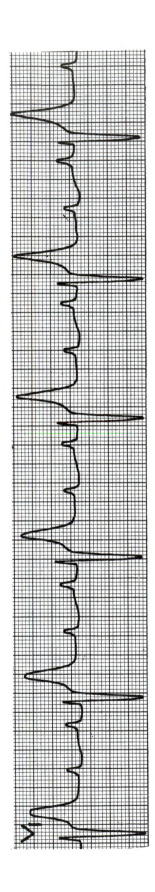

149

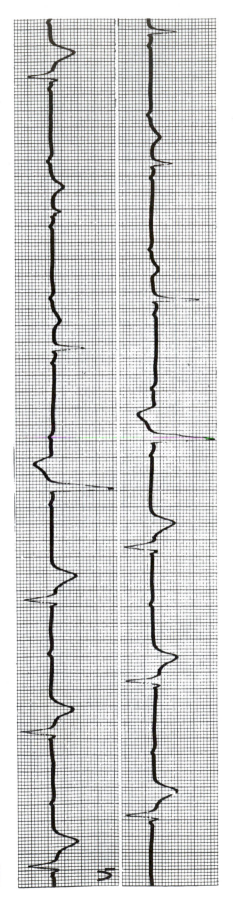

150

149 **Diagnosis. Sinus tachycardia** (rate 122/min) with probable **complete A-V block** and **idioventricular rhythm** at a rate of 41/min.

Special Points. At first glance, this looks like 3:1 A-V block. However, if one looks carefully at the P-R intervals of the apparently conducted beats, a progressive shortening by tiny decrements is detected: the first P-R is 0.29 sec and the last is 0.25 sec. This slight but steady decrease in the P-R interval is strong evidence in favor of A-V independence and therefore complete A-V block (compare Figure 89).

150 **Diagnosis. Sinus rhythm with (presumably) Type II** 2:1 **A-V block** with **LBBB**; left idioventricular escape at a rate of 36/min with frequent **fusion beats.**

Special Points. The idioventricular rhythm has a rate almost exactly half the sinus rate. Therefore, when 2:1 block is present, there is competition between the idioventricular and the conducted rhythms, producing series of fusion beats. Each strip begins with three idioventricular beats from the left ventricle, followed by a conducted beat with LBBB. In the upper strip, the next two beats are fusion beats, and the last is another idioventricular beat. In lower strip, the last three beats are all fusion beats. Because the ectopic ventricular focus is on the same side as the bundle-branch block, simultaneous activation of both ventricles narrows and normalizes the fusion complexes. As Schamroth neatly puts it, "Two wrongs sometimes make a right!" Several other examples of this are shown in the Red Zone.

151

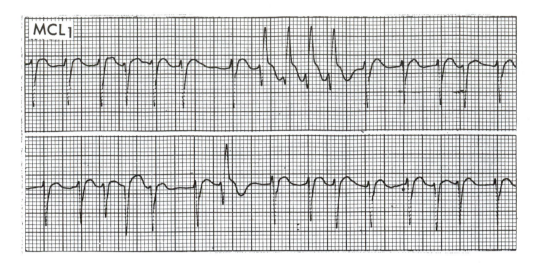

152

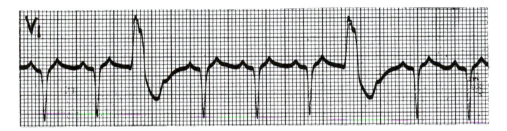

153

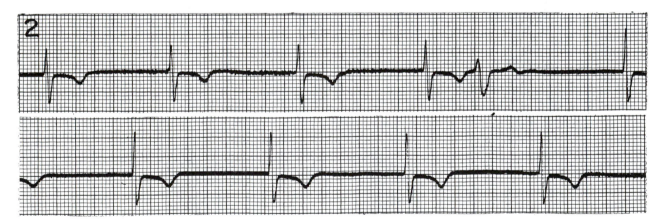

151

Diagnosis. **Atrial fibrillation** with rapid ventricular response (about 175/min) and a run of **RBBB aberration** precipitated by the lengthened ventricular cycle. In the bottom strip there is one aberrantly conducted beat.

Special Points. Note the classic triphasic rSR′ pattern of the aberrant beats. When a relatively long cycle is followed by a relatively short cycle that ends with aberrant conduction, it is known as the Ashman phenomenon.

Treatment. The aberration itself requires no treatment. If runs of aberrant beats are mistaken for ventricular tachycardia, lidocaine or another antiarrhythmic agent may be given with unfortunate results: the ventricular rate may increase dangerously. Proper treatment, regardless of whether the anomalous beats are aberrant or ectopic, is aimed at the primary disturbance: atrial fibrillation with a rapid ventricular response. The ventricular response should be slowed with digitalis, propranolol, or verapamil or the arrhythmia terminated by electrical cardioversion.

152

Diagnosis. **Atrial tachycardia** (rate 212/min) with 2:1 conduction; two left **VPBs.**

Special Points. The anomalous beats are identified as ventricular ectopic by their early peak (taller left rabbit ear) and by their width of 0.16 sec.

Note also that a preceding P wave does not necessarily imply conduction to the ensuing QRS complex.

Treatment. Efforts should first be aimed at restoring a normal ventricular rate, for which digitalis, propranolol, or verapamil would be appropriate, depending on the clinical circumstances.

153

Diagnosis. **Sick sinus syndrome** (no evidence of atrial activity) with **junctional rhythm** at 45/min; one **VPB** with **concealed retrograde conduction** into the A-V junction.

Special Point. The cycle after the VPB is as long as the junctional escape cycles, indicating that the junctional pacemaker has been depolar-

ized and reset by retrograde conduction from the VPB (see laddergram).

Treatment. If the patient is asymptomatic, no treatment is indicated. If the sick sinus syndrome is producing symptoms, then a permanent pacemaker is probably indicated, provided that the patient is not receiving drugs (e.g., propranolol) that could account for the ailing sinus.

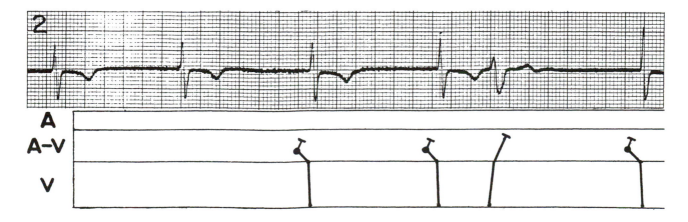

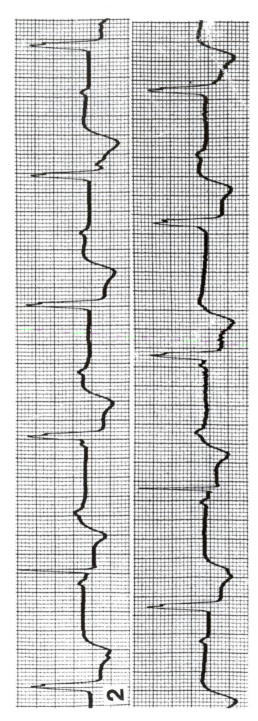

154

154

Diagnosis. Sinus rhythm with **some degree of A-V block, idioventricular escape rhythm** at rate of 44/min with two **ventricular captures** (see laddergram). (Morphology of the captured beats suggests left ventricular hypertrophy with superimposed myocardial ischemia.) Tracing courtesy of Dr. David Spodick.

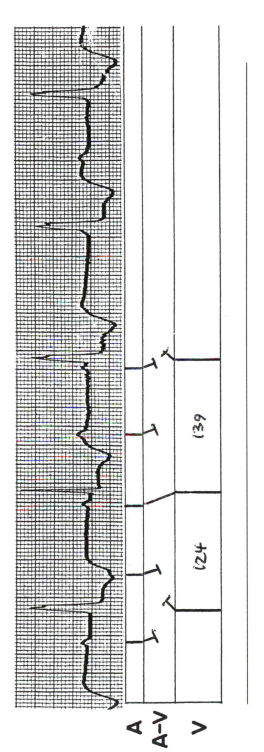

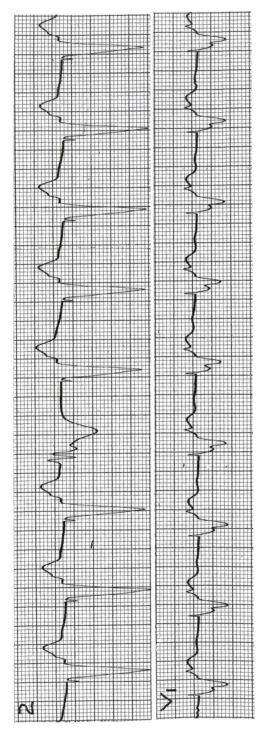

155

2

V₁

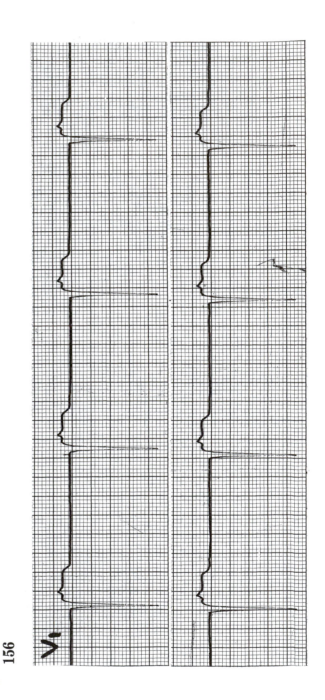

156

V₁

155

Diagnosis. Right ventricular demand pacemaker (rate 72/min) interrupted by one appropriately sensed **VPB**; all the paced beats are conducted retrogradely to the atria.

156

Diagnosis. Sick sinus permitting junctional escape rhythm at rate of 37/min with retrograde conduction to atria.

157

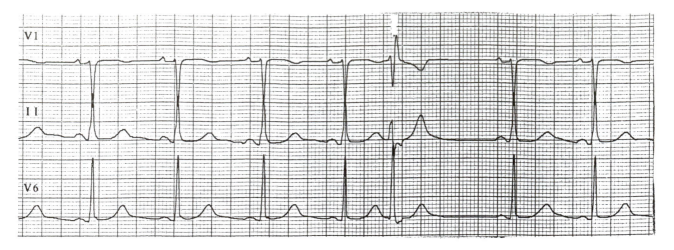

158

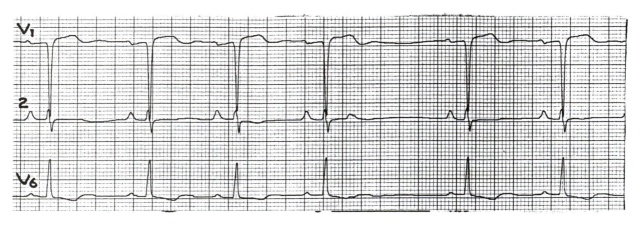

159

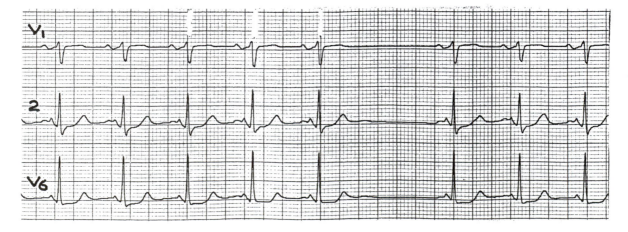

157

Diagnosis. Sinus rhythm interrupted by a **junctional premature beat** with **RBBB aberration** and retrograde conduction to atria.

158

Diagnosis. Sinus rhythm interrupted by **nonconducted APB**.

159

Diagnosis. **Type II S-A block.**

Special Point. The most likely explanation for a sudden unexpected pause is always a nonconducted APB. However, here there is no visible evidence of premature atrial activity, the P-P intervals of the shorter cycles are all the same, and the unexpected long cycle equals two of the short cycles. Therefore, Type II S-A block is the preferred diagnosis.

160

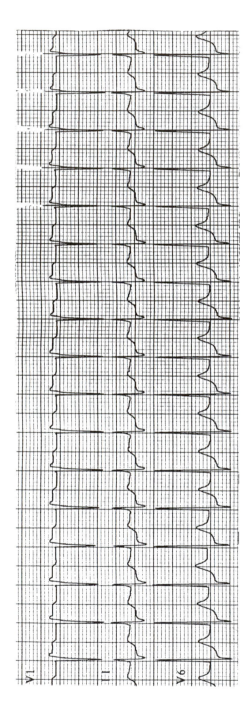

V1

II

V6

161

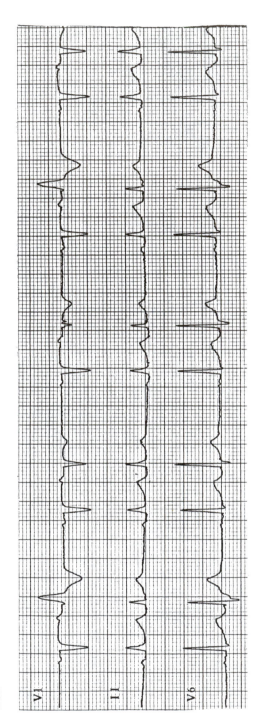

V1

II

V6

160

Diagnosis. **A-V nodal reentrant tachycardia** (rate 150/min).

Special Point. There is no definite recognizable atrial activity; therefore, the working diagnosis is AVNRT. Of course the terminal r in V_1 and s in lead 2 and V_6 may be "pseudo-r" and "pseudo-s" waves, representing the tail end of retrograde atrial activity—in which case the diagnosis of AVNRT is confirmed.

161

Diagnosis. Sinus rhythm with **atrial bigeminy** showing varying degrees of **RBBB aberration.**

Special Point. Note that the earliest signs of RBB delay, that is, shrinkage of S wave and slurring or notching of the terminal part of the S wave, are well seen in V_1 in the QRSs of the second and third APBs.

162

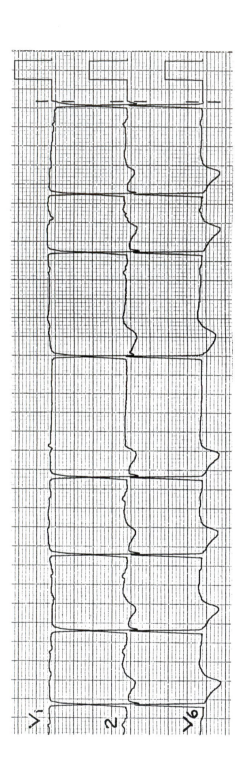

V₁

2

V₆

163

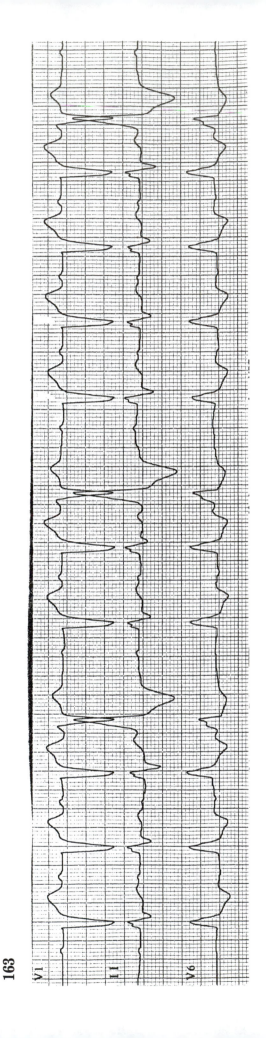

V1

II

V6

162

Diagnosis. Sinus rhythm with mild **first-degree A-V block** (P-R = 0.22 sec), interrupted by two **APBs**, the first nonconducted and followed by junctional escape. (The QRS-T pattern suggests left ventricular enlargement.)

163

Diagnosis. Sinus rhythm with **first-degree A-V block** (P-R = 0.30 sec) and LBBB interrupted by three **right VPBs.**

164

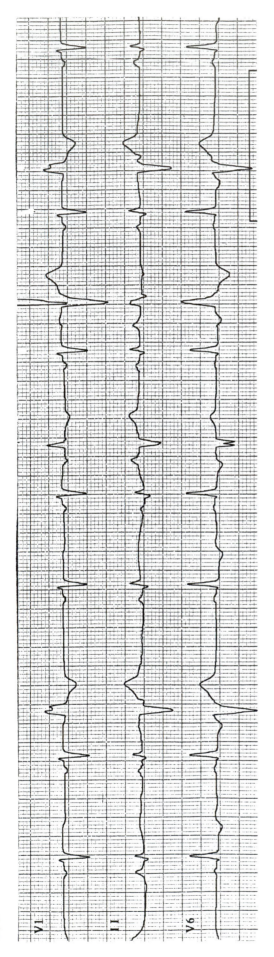

V1

II

V6

165

2

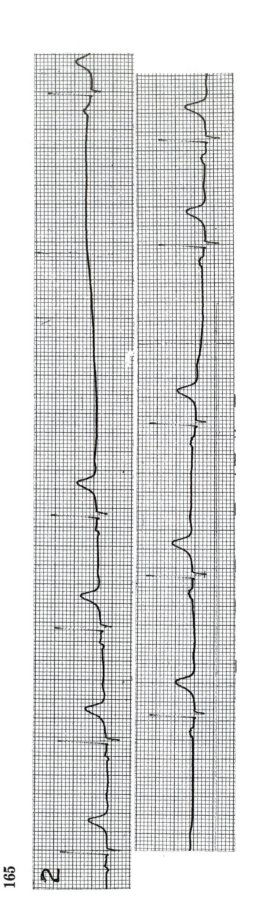

164

Diagnosis. Sinus bradycardia (rate 56/min) is interrupted first by a left **VPB** and then, three beats later, by an **APB** with apparent aberrant ventricular conduction, but because the morphology of this QRS is unlike any recognizable conduction pattern and because the polarity in each lead is identical with that of the previous VPB, it is more likely that this is a fusion beat between another VPB from that focus and the APB. Two beats later there is another APB with LBBB aberration and then finally another left VPB with retrograde conduction to the atria.

165

Diagnosis. A sick sinus syndrome. An ectopic atrial rhythm at rate 50/min stops abruptly, and after 4.5 sec the sinus finally escapes and gradually accelerates from a rate of 31–56/min.

166

V1

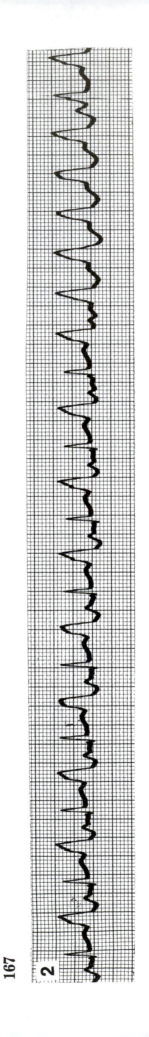

167

2

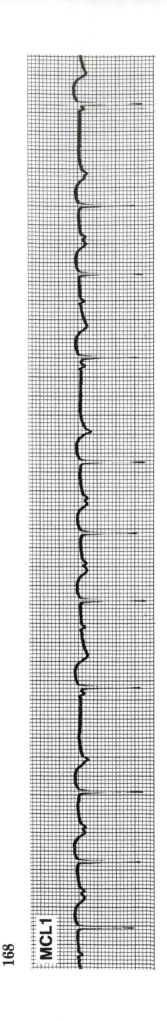

168

MCL1

166

Diagnosis. Sinus rhythm with **first-degree A-V block** and **RBBB**, twice interrupted by **nonconducted APBs**.

Special Point. The first P-R in each group is somewhat shorter than the subsequent P-Rs, and so the first QRS in each group may be a junctional escape beat or it may simply be an expression of R-P:P-R reciprocity typical of A-V nodal block.

167

Diagnosis. Sinus rhythm with **interpolated ventricular bigeminy**; after the ninth sinus beat, **ventricular tachycardia** develops and the penultimate beat is a **fusion beat**. (The sinus beat reveal the underlying lesion: acute inferior infarction).

168

Diagnosis. **Type I second-degree A-V block** with Wenckebach periods; after each "dropped" beat, the returning beat is a **junctional escape**.

169

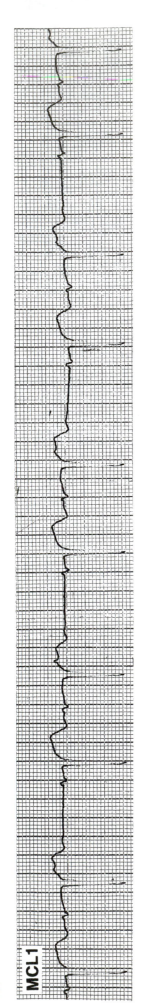

MCL1

170

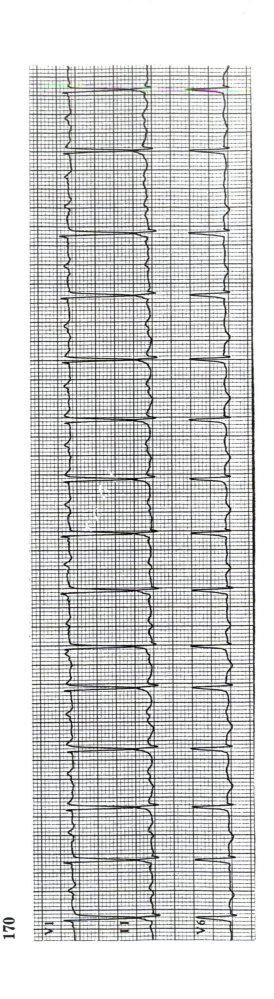

171

2

169

Diagnosis. Potential **Type I A-V block**; Wenckebach-type conduction is interrupted by **nonconducted APBs**, leaving the QSRs grouped in pairs.

Special Point. The QRS-T configuration looks like an anteroseptal infarction—which is not usually associated with Type I A-V block; however, this could be an inferior infarction because when an *inferior* infarction is associated with *right* ventricular involvement—as it often is—the ST segment in V_1 (or MCL_1) may be elevated.

170

Diagnosis. **Atrial tachycardia** (rate 192/min) with varying AV conduction.

171

Diagnosis. **Ventricular tachycardia** (rate 160/min), with frequent **fusion beats.**

Special Point. Note the independent P waves; 1st, 7th, 13th, and 19th beats are ventricular fusion beats.

172

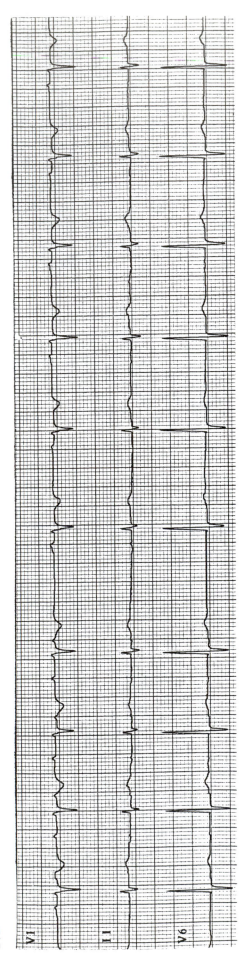

V1

II

V6

173

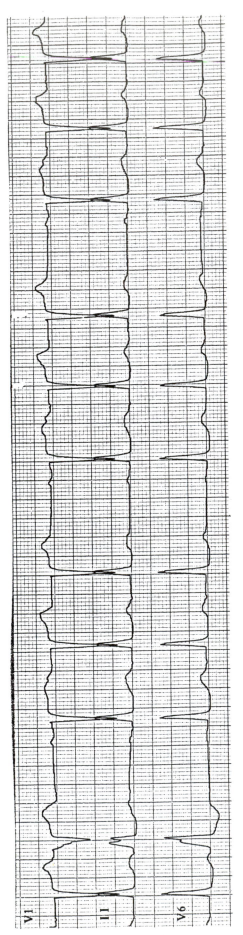

V1

II

V6

172

Diagnosis. **Atrial tachycardia** at rate 150/min abruptly stops just after the fourth QRS, whereupon the sinus assumes control for the rest of the strip.

173

Diagnosis. Sinus rhythm with **Type I A-V block** producing **4:3 Wenckebach periods**; one right VPB.

Special Point. In the VPB, note the typical slurred downstroke to a delayed (more than 0.07 sec) nadir; compare with the slick downstroke and early nadir (less than 0.07 sec) of LBBB.

174

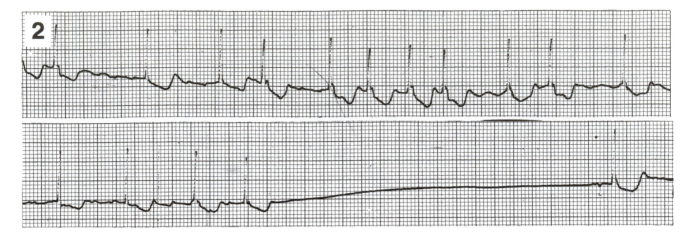

175

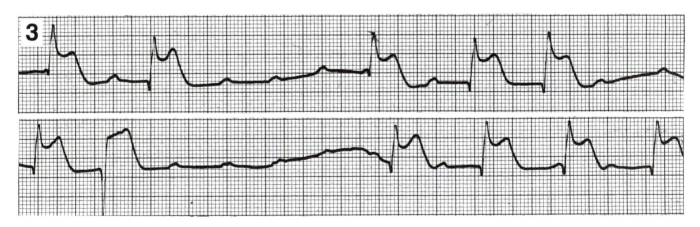

176

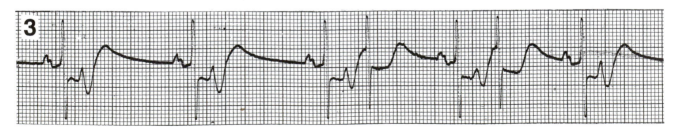

174

Diagnosis. **Tachycardia-bradycardia (sick sinus) syndrome.**

Special Point. An irregular tachyarrhythmia suddenly ceases and after a long, silent pause the junction escapes. (The ST-T pattern suggests digitalis effect).

175

Diagnosis. **Sinus tachycardia** with **high-grade**, Type I A-V block in a patient with acute inferior infarction; **one VPB**.

176

Diagnosis. Sinus rhythm with conducted and nonconducted **APBs**.

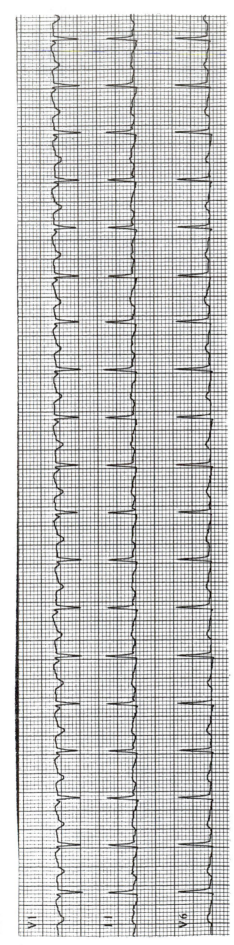

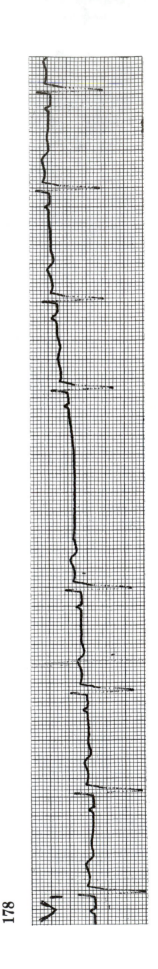

177

178

177

Diagnosis. Atrial tachycardia (rate 240/min) with **2:1 A-V conduction.**

Special Point. Notice avoidance of the term "2:1 **block.**" This is because "block" connotes abnormality, and there is nothing abnormal in an A-V node refusing to transmit 240 impulses/min; moreover, the diagnosis of 2:1 block has a malignant ring to many ears.

In the supraventricular tachycardias, 2:1 conduction is notoriously difficult to recognize. This is because with 2:1 conduction, one of the atrial waves is inevitably synchronous with some part of the ventricular complex, and therefore it is rare to get two distinctly recognizable atrial waves between QSRs. This is particularly true at atrial rates diagnosable as atrial flutter (see Figure 182).

178

Diagnosis. Sinus bradycardia with **Type II S-A block**; one APB.

Special Point. The P-P intervals preceding the dropped beat are all the same, and the cycle of the dropped beat is equal to two of the shorter cycles.

179

2

180

V₁

181

V6

179

Diagnosis. The combination of **sinus arrhythmia** and **A-V block** produces a form of **escape-capture bigeminy**; the first beat of each pair is a junctional escape and the second of each pair is a ventricular capture with prolonged P-R interval.

180

Diagnosis. **Sinus arrhythmia** with **rate-dependent LBBB**.

181

Diagnosis. **Sinus bradycardia** with normal P-R interval, **RBBB**, and **high-grade A-V block.** Four consecutive blocked beats result in **ventricular asystole** for 7 sec and confirm the probability that the block is infranodal (Type II).

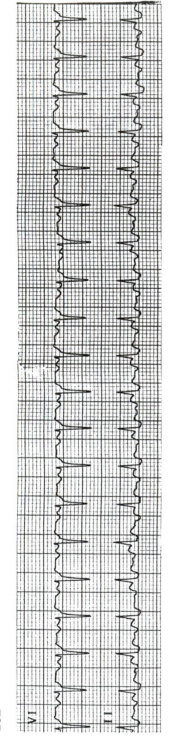

182

V1

II

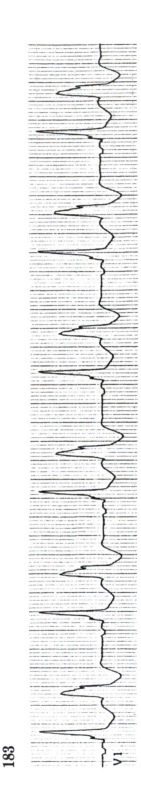

183

V1

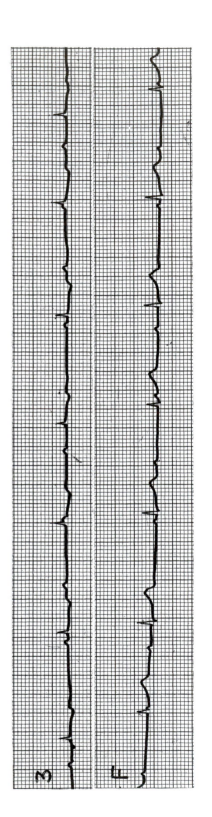

184

3

F

182

Diagnosis. **Atrial flutter** (rate 304/min) with **2:1 A-V conduction.**

183

Diagnosis. Sinus rhythm with **RBBB** and **left ventricular bigeminy.**

Special Point. Note that the VPBs have typical ectopic morphology with left peak taller than right.

184

Diagnosis. A-V dissociation between sinus rhythm (rate 90/min) and **junctional escape rhythm** (rate 52/min) because of **Type I A-V block.** Fourth and seventh beats in the top strip and second and fifth beats in bottom strip are **ventricular captures.**

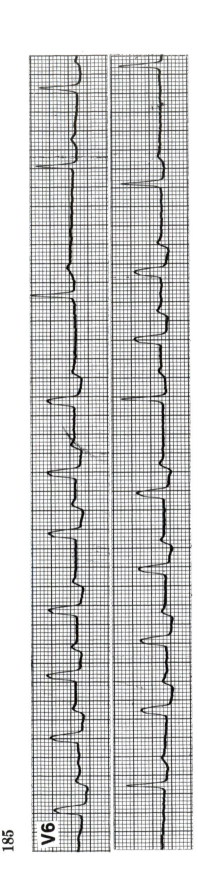

185

V6

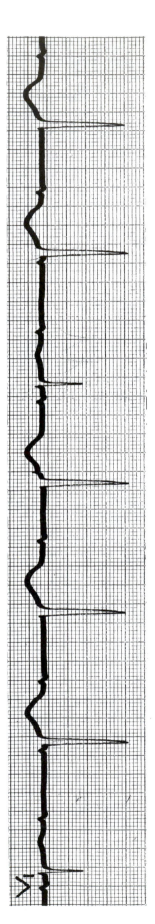

186

V1

185

Diagnosis. **Atrial fibrillation** with rate-dependent **LBBB**.

186

Diagnosis. Sinus rhythm with (probable) **Type I** (narrow QSRs, no BBB) **A-V block** with resulting **idioventricular escape** at 45/min; fifth beat is **ventricular capture.**

Special Point. Despite the normal P-R, the absence of BBB makes the level of block most likely A-V nodal.

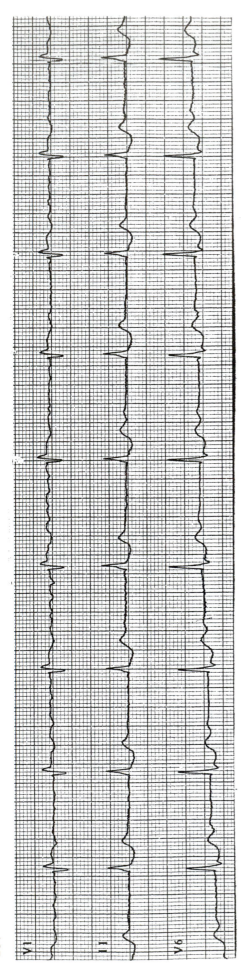

187

Diagnosis. **Atrial fibrillation** with some degree of **A-V block** permitting **junctional escape** at 54/min; **incomplete RBBB; questionable digitalis effect.**

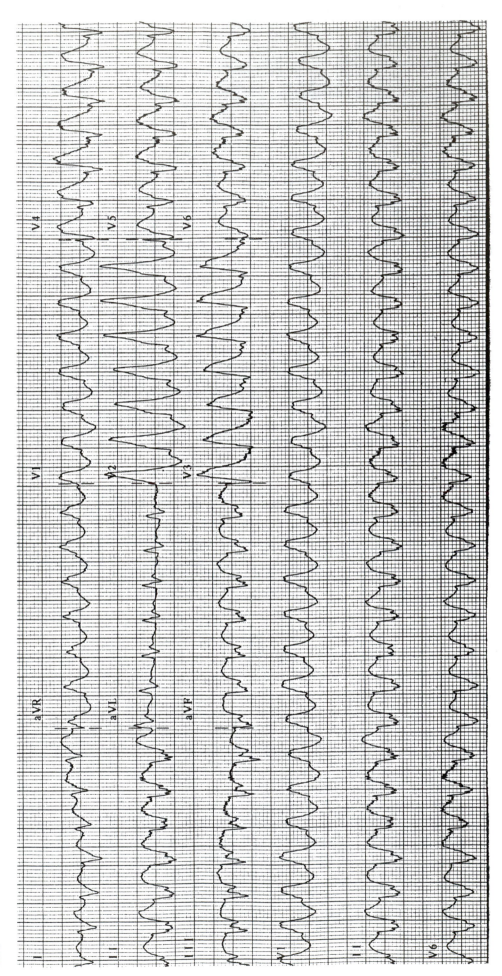

188

188

Diagnosis. Left ventricular tachycardia.

Special Point. Clues favoring ventricular tachycardia are axis in "no man's land," rS in V_6. Note also that a preexcited tachycardia (WPW) is excluded by the negative QRSs, V_{4-6} and the qR in V_3.[a]

---

[a]Steurer, G., Gursoy, S., Frey, B., et al.: The differential diagnosis on the electrocardiogram between ventricular tachycardia and preexcited tachycardia. Clin. Cardiol. *17*:306, 1994.

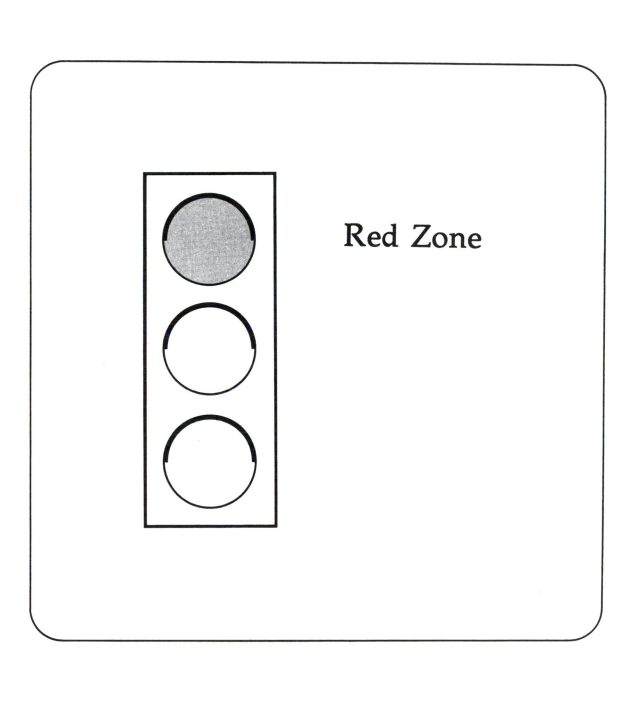

Red Zone

189

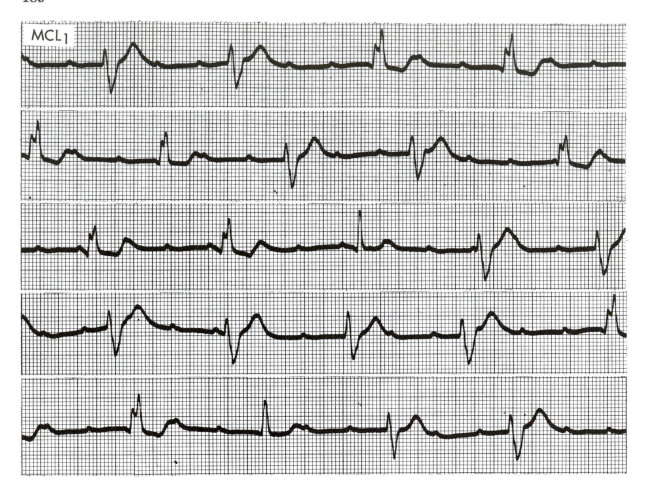

189

Diagnosis. **Sinus tachycardia** (rate 135/min) with **complete A-V block,** competing idioventricular pacemakers, one in each ventricle, and resulting **ventricular fusion beats.**

Special Point. This is the second situation (compare Figure 138) in which fusion beats, because they are produced by simultaneous activation of the two ventricles, are narrower than either of the component complexes. Here, both pacemakers have similar rates of 40–50/min, but because of the slight irregularity of both, it is impossible to be sure of all the fusion beats. However, the following beats are definitely fusions: second beat in second strip, third beat in third strip, and second and third beats in bottom strip.

190

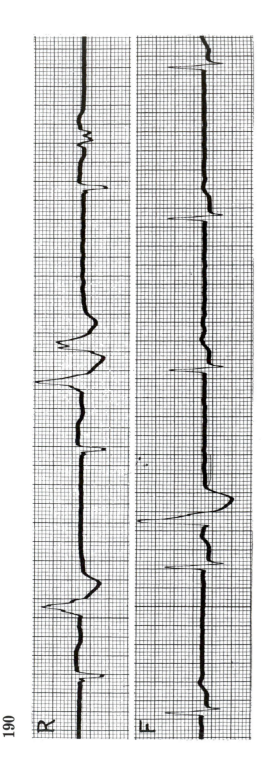

191

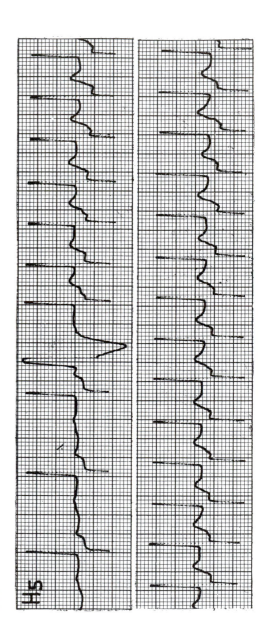

190

Diagnosis. **Atrial fibrillation** with **complete A-V block** and **idiojunctional rhythm** at a rate of 37/min; frequent **multifocal VPBs,** including one pair, with **concealed retrograde conduction** into the junction.

Special Point. Because the VPBs are followed by a cycle approximately equal to the independent junctional cycle, it is obvious that the premature ventricular impulses have discharged the junctional pacemaker and reset its rhythm. Because this retrograde conduction can be inferred only by its effect on the next beat (resetting of the junctional rhythm), it qualifies as "concealed" conduction.

191

Diagnosis. **Sinus rhythm with first-degree A-V block** interrupted by a **VPB** that initiates **reentrant A-V nodal tachycardia.**

Special Point. All that is needed to initiate a reentrant A-V nodal tachycardia is for an impulse to enter the A-V node and find a circuit ripe for reentry. This is usually achieved by a premature atrial impulse that finds the fast pathway still refractory after the slow pathway has recovered, so the APB is conducted with a prolonged P-R interval, and reentry is established. Because it is common for ventricular ectopic impulses to be conducted retrogradely into the junction, and indeed all the way to the atria, it is not surprising that an occasional VPB finds a ready circuit in the node and initiates a reentrant tachycardia.

192

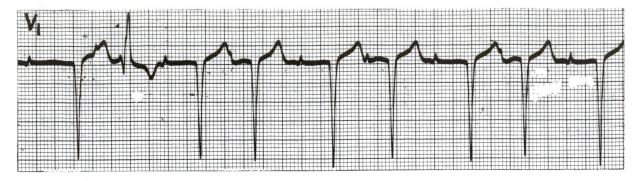

192

Diagnosis. **Sinus rhythm with alternating prolonged P-R intervals, most likely due to concealed junctional extrasystoles** occurring every third beat (see laddergram); the second sinus impulse is conducted with **RBBB aberration.** (The QRS-T pattern is that of left ventricular hypertrophy.)

Special Point. The R-P/P-R relationship is not reciprocal as one would expect; with the shorter R-P interval, one would expect a longer P-R, and vice versa. But here the shorter R-P is complemented by a shorter P-R, and the longer R-P by a longer P-R. Because the atrial impulse ending the shorter R-P is conducted better than would be expected, it was assumed to be due to "supernormal" conduction until Langendorf,[a] in a classic paper, postulated the influence of concealed junctional extrasystoles. It was not until more than two decades later that the validity of his explanation was proved by His bundle electrography.

Because you cannot see concealed junctional extrasystoles in the clinical tracing, their diagnosis is always by inference—until the patient gets to the electrophysiology lab. But junctional extrasystoles should always come to mind under three circumstances: (1) when there is sudden unexplained lengthening of a P-R interval, (2) when one sees Type II A-V conduction behavior in the absence of BBB, and (3) when Type I and Type II block appear to coexist in the same tracing. In any of these circumstances, suspicion is supported by the finding of manifest junctional extrasystoles elsewhere in the tracing.

---

[a] Langendorf, R., and Mehlman, J. S.: Blocked (nonconducted) A-V nodal premature systoles imitating first and second degree A-V block. Am. Heart J. *34*:500, 1947.

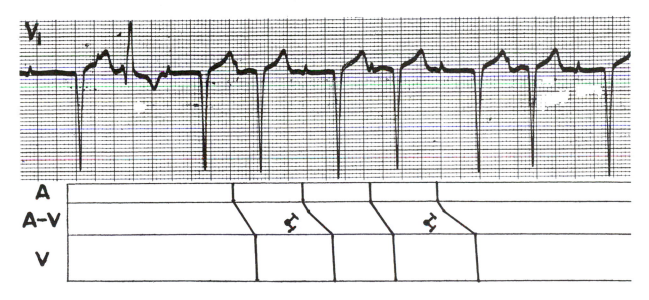

193

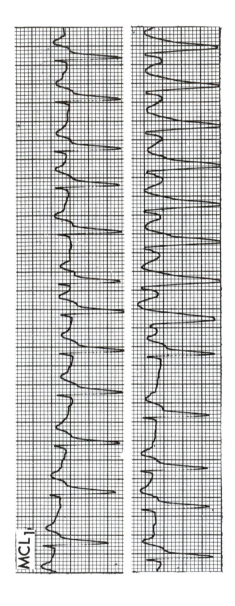

MCL₁

194

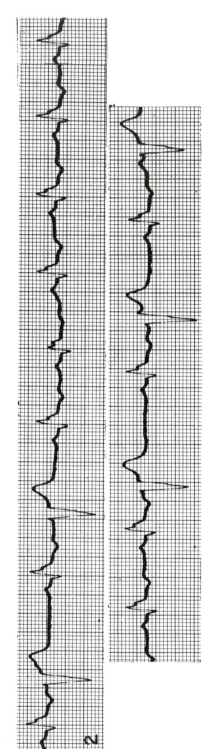

2

193

Diagnosis. Atrial fibrillation with rapid ventricular response (rate about 126/min) and **LBBB.** In the middle of the bottom strip, a right VPB initiates **ventricular tachycardia** (rate 146/min).

Special Point. On casual inspection, it may appear that the LBBB has increased in the middle of the bottom strip; however, the simultaneous development of absolute regularity and the tell-tale widening of the initial R wave[a] indicate right ventricular tachycardia.

[a] Swanick, E. J., LaCamera, F., Jr., and Marriott, H. J. L.: Morphologic features of right ventricular ectopic beats. Am. J. Cardiol. 30:888, 1972.

194

Diagnosis. Sinus rhythm with RBBB; ventricular parasystole with one **fusion beat.** (The QRS complexes reveal the underlying acute inferior infarction.)

Special Points. This is a beautiful example of parasystole. One first notices that the coupling intervals of the ectopic beats are quite variable, and this immediately brings to mind a parasystolic mechanism. If calipers are then set to the interectopic interval at the beginning of the

top strip (177) and that interval is marched through the remainder of the tracing, one first lands on the sixth beat, which is a fusion beat (F), and then either at points where the ventricles are refractory or exactly where subsequent ectopic beats appear (see intervals in figure). This proves an independent undisturbable rhythm—like a fixed-rate pacemaker—and that is parasystole. Remembering that a fixed-rate pacemaker is the perfect artificial analogue of parasystole makes the diagnosis of parasystole easy.

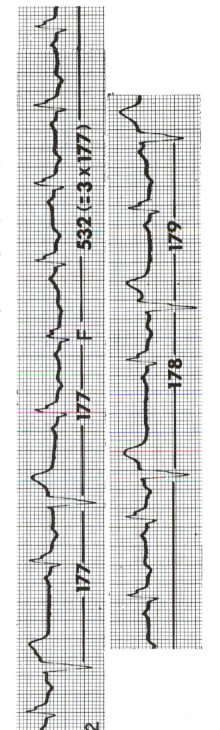

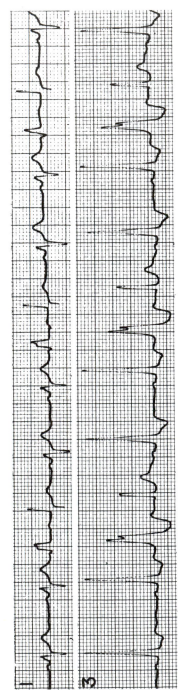

195

3

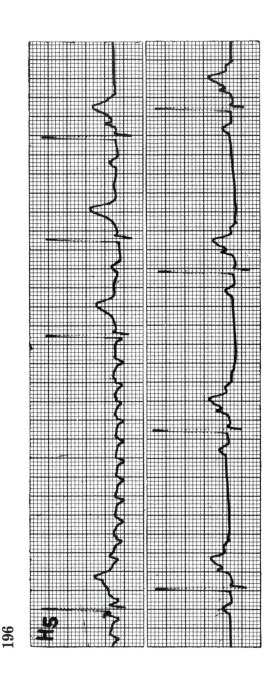

196

H5

195

Diagnosis. Sinus rhythm with preexcitation (Wolff-Parkinson-White syndrome) interrupted by frequent **VPBs** with **concealed retrograde conduction** into the accessory pathway.

Special Point. After each VPB, the P-R interval of the next sinus beat lengthens while its QRS complex narrows. This indicates that the accessory pathway has been temporarily blocked, presumably the aftereffect of concealed retrograde conduction from the VPBs.

196

Diagnosis. Top strip: end of a paroxysm of atrial flutter with considerable **concealed conduction** into the A-V junction; **sinus bradycardia** with **first-degree A-V block** and R-P–dependent P-R intervals; one **nonconducted APB.** Bottom strip: sinus rhythm with first-degree A-V block (P-R interval = 0.24 sec) with paired nonconducted APBs.

Special Points. Remember that in the presence of atrial fibrillation or atrial flutter, there is often considerable concealed conduction into the junction, making the A-V block look much worse than it is. Here, for instance, during the atrial flutter, it looks as though there is considerable A-V block, yet the last two beats in the top strip demonstrate that the patient is capable of conducting every beat with only first-degree A-V block when the atrial rate is 56/min.

The slow sinus rate revealed at the end of the top strip may be temporary and due to overdrive suppression by the atrial flutter.

Treatment. In this situation, treatment should be aimed at eliminating the atrial arrhythmia rather than at the A-V block.

197

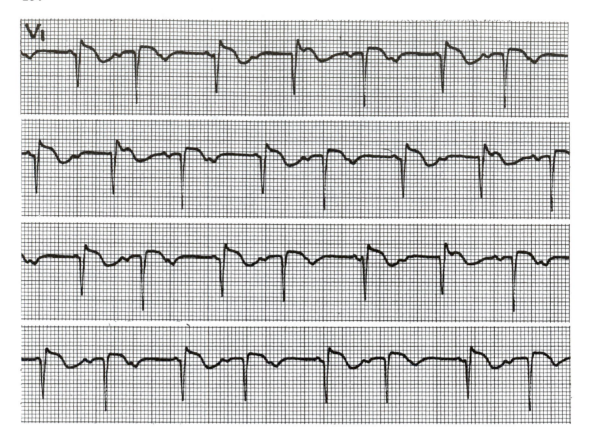

197

Diagnosis. Sinus tachycardia (rate 122/min) with some degree of **A-V block,** combined with an **accelerated junctional rhythm** at a rate of 74/min, producing **A-V dissociation** ("block-acceleration dissociation"), with every second or third beat a **ventricular capture** with slightly prolonged P-R intervals; **incomplete RBBB aberration** of the junctional beats.

Special Points. This relatively mild manifestation of A-V block is often overdiagnosed as high-grade block because most of the atrial impulses are not conducted. To appreciate the mildness of the block, merely observe the cycle of the capture beats and the rate that that cycle represents (in this case about 96/min). One can then confidently say that if only the atrial rate were 96 instead of 122, every beat would be conducted with a little first-degree block. Let me reemphasize the important fact that with a slightly ailing A-V node, an increase in the atrial rate is a serious handicap to conduction (compare similar situations in Figures 221 and 224).

The pattern of the junctional beats suggests that they originate in a focus on the left side of the His bundle so that they are preferentially conducted down the left bundle branch, producing slight comparative delay in right ventricular activation (see diagram). This is sometimes called Type B aberration, that is, ventricular aberration that is secondary to abnormal conduction above the ventricles. The various mechanisms that can cause this form of aberration are illustrated in the diagram: eccentric site of the junctional pacemaker, causing preferential conduction down the ipsilateral bundle branch and therefore the pattern of delayed conduction in the contralateral branch (1); deflection of the descending impulse by an area of nonconducting, diseased tissue favoring conduction down the contralateral branch (2); conduction to the ventricles via a paraspecific (Mahaim) tract (3); and A-V conduction via an accessory pathway (4).

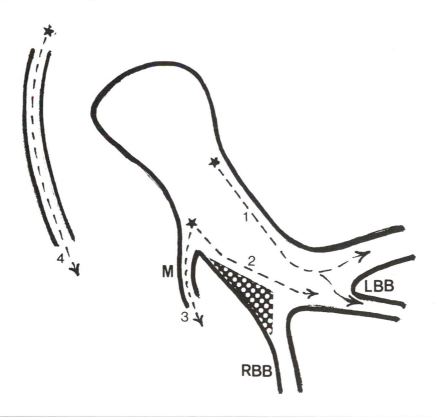

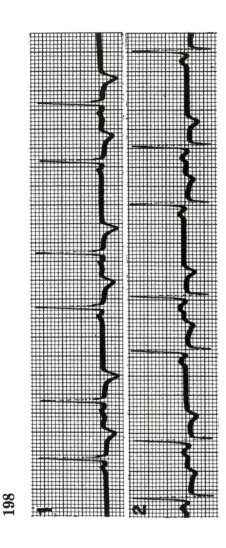

198

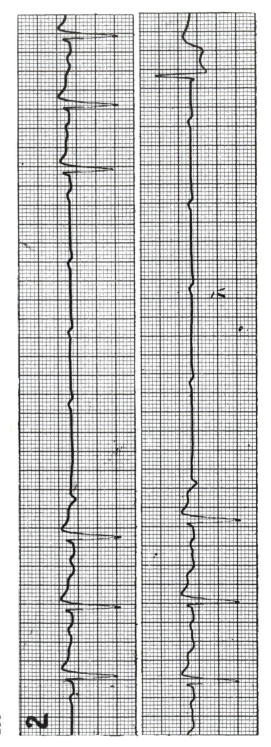

199

198

Diagnosis. Sinus tachycardia (rate 110/min) with 3 : 2 **Wenckebach** periods out of the sinus node (see laddergram).

Special Point. Whenever you see identical P waves—or for that matter identical QRS complexes—deployed in pairs, always consider 3 : 2 Wenckebach conduction first.

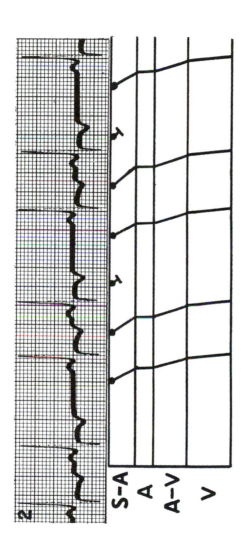

199

Diagnosis. Sinus rhythm with **first-degree A-V block** (P-R interval = 0.24 sec) interrupted by **nonconducted APBs**, which in each strip precipitate A-V block; this in turn is complicated by **ventricular asystole** for several seconds. The bottom strip ends with a single **ventricular escape beat.**

Special Point. The explanation for APBs precipitating A-V block is uncertain. It is often attributed to the same mechanism that produces paradoxical aberration, that is, block that develops only after longer cycles. In situations such as that depicted here, the APB—by "overdrive suppression"—lengthens the interval before conduction is again attempted (next sinus P wave). This, however, fails to explain why conduction again resumes after an even much longer cycle.

200

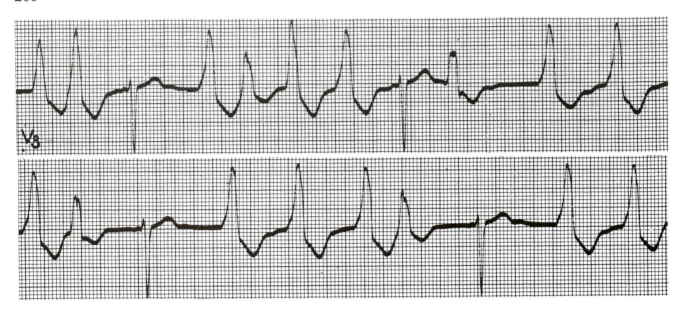

200

Diagnosis. **Sinus rhythm interrupted by ventricular extrasystoles** and **parasystole.**

Special Point. The key to solving this arrhythmia is the pair of ectopic beats at the end of each strip. If calipers are set at the interval represented by these pairs and marched backward, one lands on each of the complexes labeled "P" (216 = 72 × 3); these are therefore parasystolic beats. Because the discharge rate of the parasystolic focus is 83/min, we are dealing with a parasystolic accelerated idioventricular rhythm.

The other ectopic beats are presumably extrasystolic (VPBs).

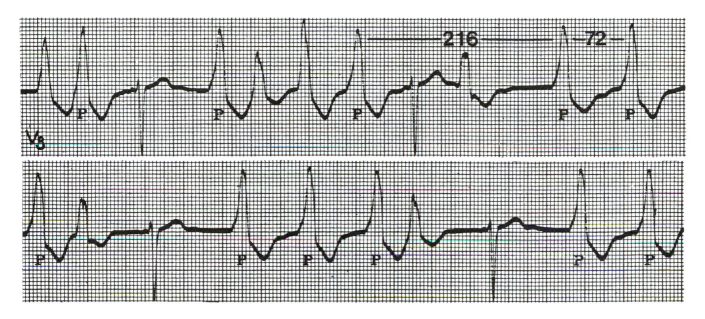

201

MCL₁

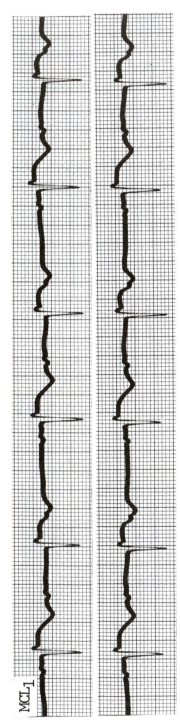

201

Diagnosis. Type I A-V block. There are two possible variants (see laddergrams): (1) a straightforward **3:2 A-V Wenckebach,** with the second conducted beat showing a remarkable increment (from 0.20 to 0.56 sec), or (2) the beats with the long P-R intervals that end the shorter ventricular cycles (which are undoubtedly conducted) may be the only conducted beats, those ending the longer cycles being **junctional escape beats.**

The QRS complexes all show the terminal r wave of incomplete RBBB.

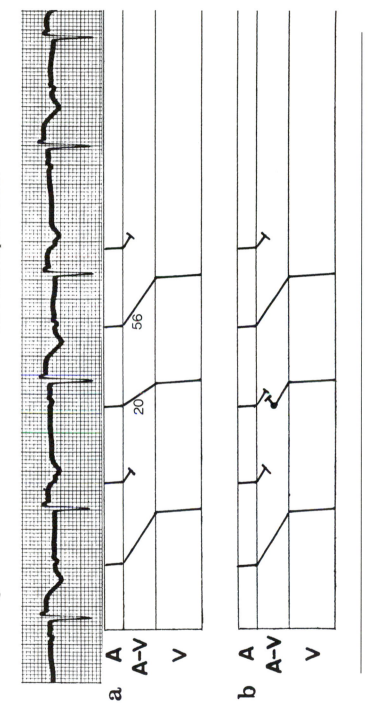

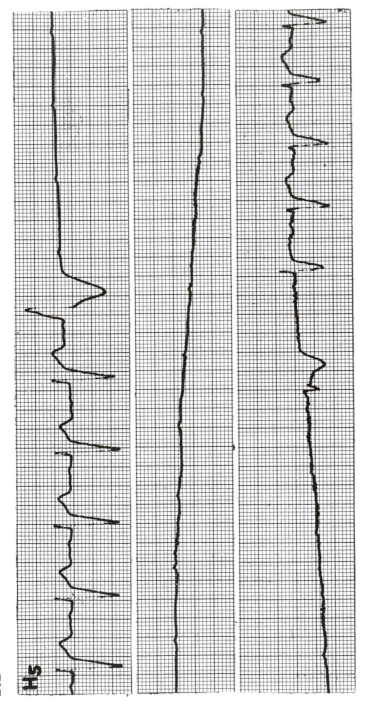

202

202

Diagnosis. **Sinus rhythm with probable RBBB** and **left anterior hemiblock; VPB** precipitating **A-V block** and **ventricular asystole.** In the bottom strip, a **ventricular escape beat** apparently restores conduction of sinus rhythm.

Special Point. Compare with Figure 152. The mechanism whereby premature beats inhibit A-V conduction is not certain, but it may be re-lated to the phenomenon of block occurring only after longer cycles.

In this case, the VPB interrupts the sequence of conducted sinus beats and enforces a longer cycle before anterograde conduction can occur again. Perhaps at the end of this longer period, conduction fails for the same reason that other blocks develop only at the end of longer cycles.

203

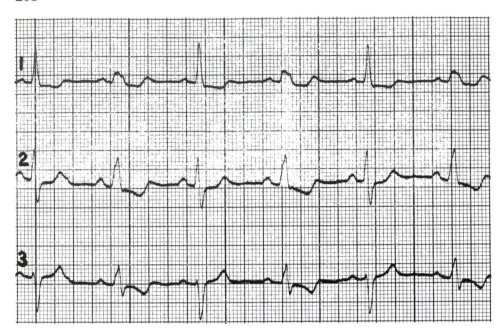

204

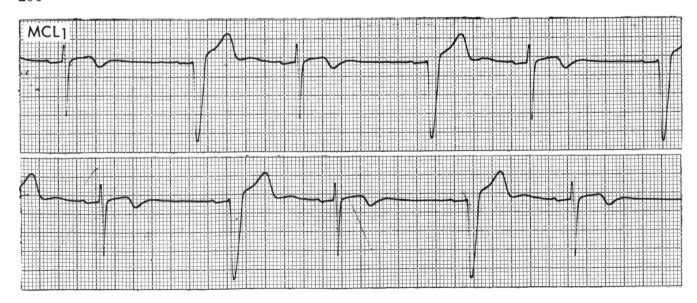

203

Diagnosis. **Sinus rhythm with alternating LBBB** and **left anterior hemiblock.**

Special Point. This sort of alternation suggests that the LBBB is postdivisional, that is, that there is constant anterior hemiblock but only 2 : 1 posterior hemiblock (see diagram).

Key: LBB = left bundle branch; a = anterior division (fascicle); p = posterior division (fascicle); LBBB = left bundle-branch block; LAHB = left anterior hemiblock.

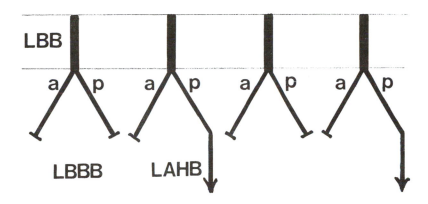

204

Diagnosis. **Sinus rhythm with 3 : 2 Wenckebach** periods out of the sinus node; **paradoxical critical rate LBBB** (also known as bradycardia-dependent LBBB).

Special Point. There are at least half a dozen theories to explain the development of BBB only at the end of longer cycles. Probably the most acceptable is that it is a phase 4 phenomenon. In brief, it is well known that as a pacemaking tissue depolarizes spontaneously (phase 4 of the action potential), it becomes more difficult for an extraneous impulse to activate it. Therefore, when block develops only with a lengthening of the cycle, it is postulated that the diseased conducting fascicle (bundle of His or bundle branch) is behaving like a pacemaker and spontaneously depolarizing. If the diseased fascicle has reached a critical stage of depolarization, the approaching sinus impulse can no longer activate it; the impulse therefore dies out and the pattern of A-V or BB block is recorded. A similar mechanism may explain the block-cum-asystole sometimes seen after an extrasystole, as in Figures 152 and 155.

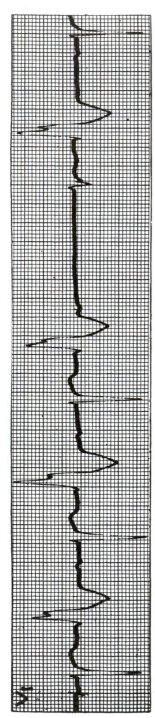

205

205

Diagnosis. **Sinus rhythm with left ventricular bigeminy; concealed retrograde conduction** from each VPB into the junction, with a progressively increasing inhibitory effect on anterograde conduction, producing a simulated A-V Wenckebach period (see laddergram); **ventricular escape.**

Special Points. Note the typical ectopic morphology, with early peak and slurring on the downstroke (taller left rabbit-ear equivalent).

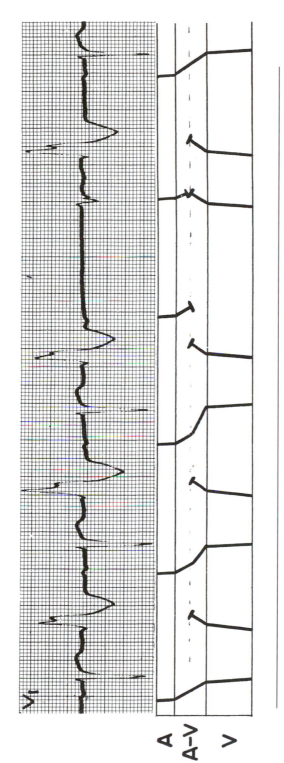

A

A–V

V

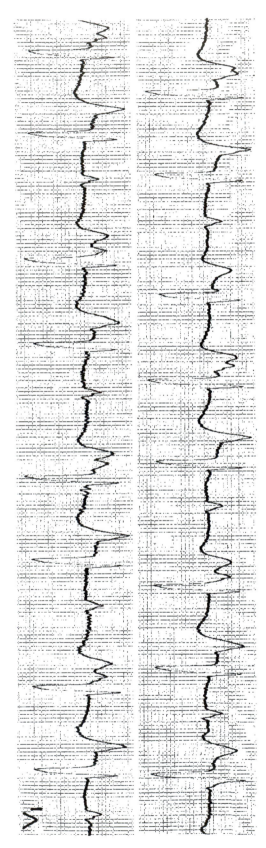

206

V1

206

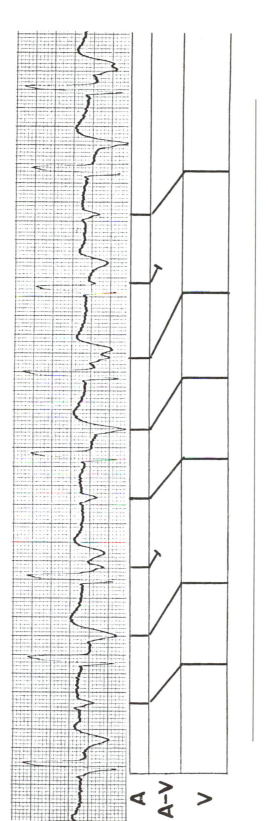

Diagnosis. Sinus rhythm with **Type I A-V block producing 3 : 2 and 4 : 3 Wenckebachs** (PR up to 0.76 sec—see laddergram); left atrial enlargement, RBBB and anteroseptal infarction of uncertain date.

207

MCL1

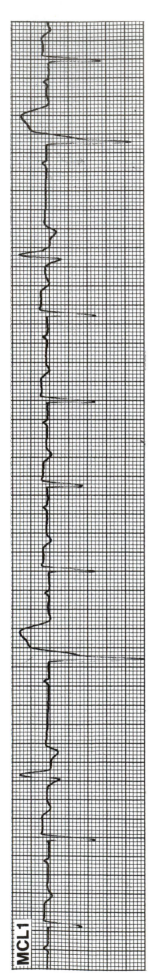

208

2

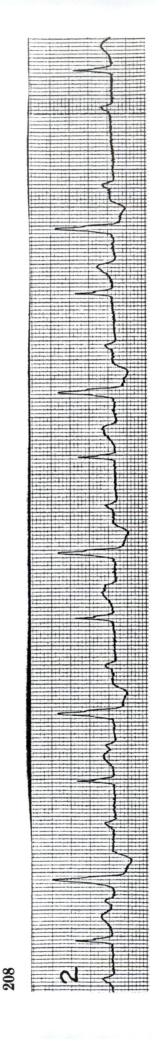

207

Diagnosis. Sinus rhythm with **first-degree A-V block** (PR = 0.24 sec) interrupted by two **VPBs**; both sinus and VPBs show pattern of anteroseptal infarction. The returning beat after each VPB is identified as supraventricular by its slick downstroke to early nadir, indicating **LBBB** rather than ventricular ectopic; they are therefore conducted sinus beats with **paradoxical (bradycardia-dependent) aberration.**

208

Diagnosis. Sinus rhythm with **first-degree A-V block** and **ventricular bigeminy; concealed retrograde conduction** from each VPB progressively lengthens the ensuing PR, producing a Wenckebach-like effect (see laddergram and compare with Figure 205).

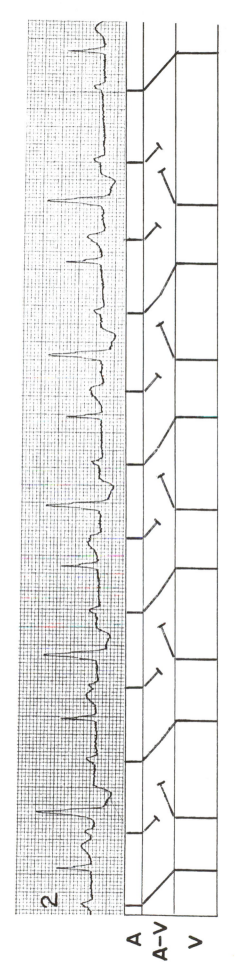

A

A–V

V

209

V1

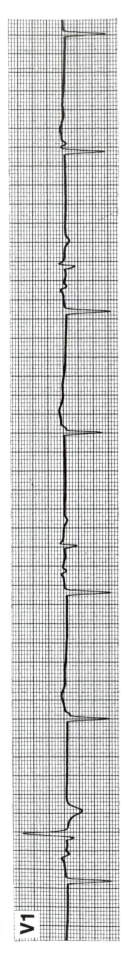

210

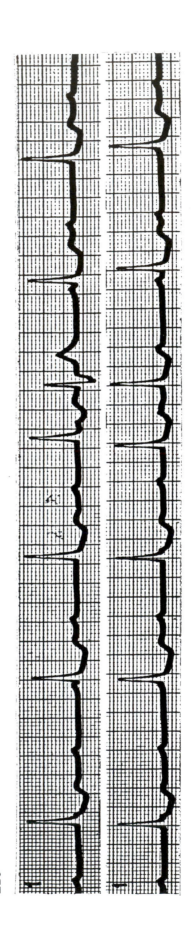

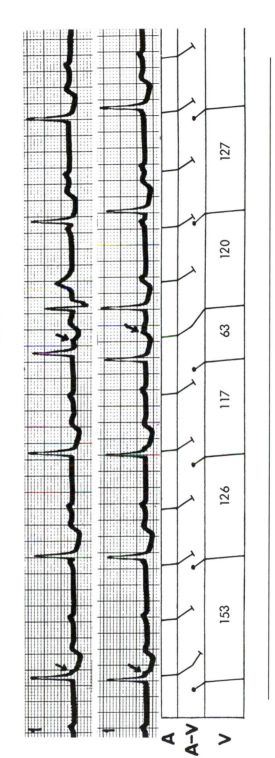

209

Diagnosis. Sinus bradycardia (rate 40/min) with **junctional escape** (rate 45/min) producing **A-V dissociation; every third beat is a ventricular capture** manifesting differing degrees of **RBBB aberration.**

210

Diagnosis. Sinus rhythm with incomplete A-V block and an independent **junctional rhythm** at a rate of 46/min. The regular junctional rhythm is interrupted by **supernormal conduction** twice in each strip: after the first beat in each strip (P wave immediately after QRS—arrow), the supernormal conduction is concealed; after the fourth beat in each strip, the supernormally conducted impulse (later P waves—arrows) reaches the ventricles, with **RBBB aberration** in the top strip.

Special Point. Remember, "supernormal" conduction is not what it says. It is not better than normal; it is better earlier than later, better than expected. Thus, in this example, one would not expect the earlier atrial impulses to be conducted when impulses later in the cycle are blocked.

A
A–V
V

153 126 117 63 120 127

211

3

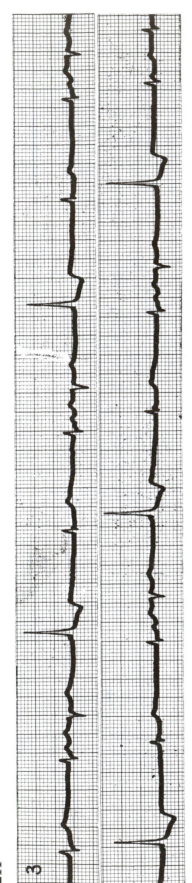

212

1

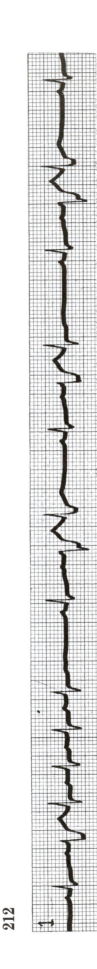

211

Diagnosis. Sinus bradycardia (rate 52/min) with **junctional** and **ventricular escape** at the respective rates of 58/min and 68/min.

Special Points. The first two beats in the top strip are junctional escapes; the second is shortly followed by a sinus impulse that is conducted, with prolonged P-R interval, to the ventricles (ventricular capture). This conducted beat is followed by a ventricular escape, which partially coincides with the next sinus P wave. The sequence—two junctional escapes, ventricular capture, ventricular escape—then repeats itself four more times. When a sequence of differing beats repeatedly recurs, it is known as an "allorhythmia."

Treatment. If any treatment is needed, it should be aimed solely at the primary, underlying disturbance, in this case, sinus bradycardia. The escape mechanisms are secondary and the prolonged P-R interval is unimportant.

212

Diagnosis. Sinus rhythm interrupted by pairs and one five-beat salvo of APBs, the first of which is always conducted with **RBBB,** and probably **left posterior hemiblock, aberration;** the 9th and 15th beats show RBBB aberration without the hemiblock. The five-beat salvo constitutes a short run of ectopic **atrial tachycardia.**

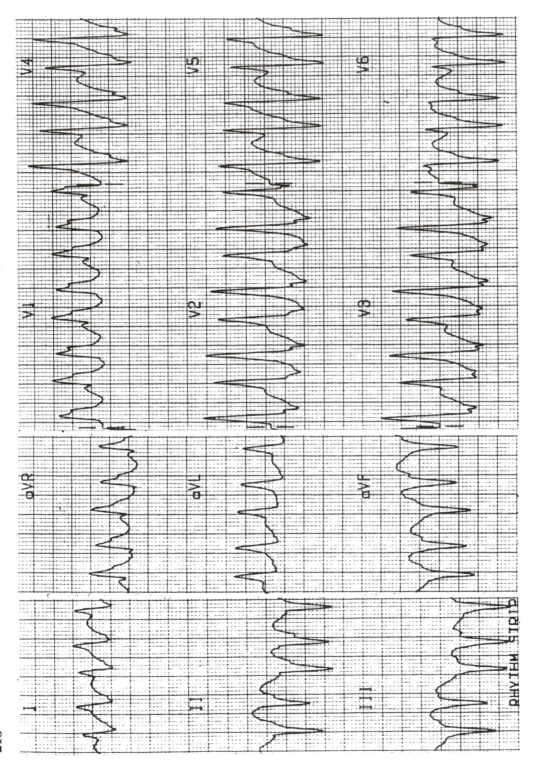

213

213

Diagnosis. Left ventricular tachycardia with 3:2 **Wenckebach** conduction out of the ectopic focus.

Special Point. The QRS morphology is entirely typical of ventricular ectopy: monophasic R wave in V_1 with taller left peak; absent q, small r, and deeper, wider S wave in V_6; and the frontal plane axis in no-man's land (about $-120°$).

The 3:2 Wenckebach exit block is presumed because the ventricular cycles alternate (longer, shorter, longer, shorter, and so on), leaving the beats in pairs.

214

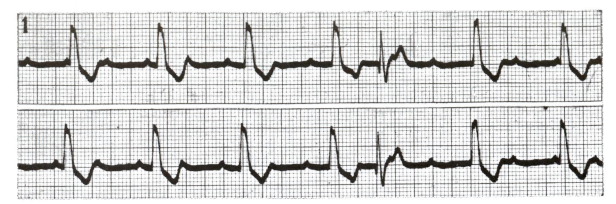

214

Diagnosis. **Some degree of A-V block** with resulting **accelerated idioventricular rhythm** producing **A-V dissociation** with two **capture beats** (thanks to **supernormal conduction**) with **RBBB.**

Special Points. This tracing is from a 47-year-old man with presumed Lenegre's disease. As usual, supernormal A-V conduction is seen only after retrograde conduction (which can reasonably be expected after the preceding idioventricular beat). Conduction qualifies as "supernormal" because it occurs when the P wave distorts the ST segment but not when it lands beyond the T wave. Thus, conduction is better than expected, better earlier than later, that is, supernormal.

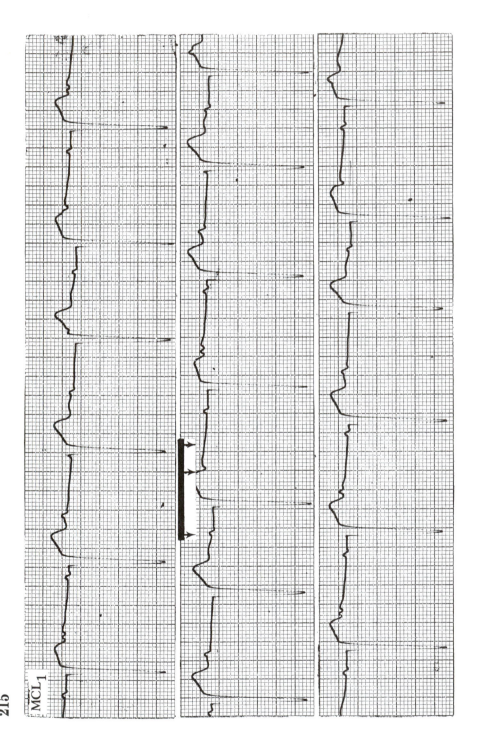

215

MCL₁

215

Diagnosis. Sinus rhythm (rate 94/min) with some degree of A-V block and consequent **junctional escape** (rate 52/min); the resulting A-V dissociation is punctuated by four **ventricular captures.** (This QRS morphology suggests left ventricular hypertrophy with probable incomplete LBBB.)

Special Points. The captured beats afford evidence of the mildness of the A-V block (they are recognized by the fact that they end cycles shorter than the junctional escape cycles, namely, the fifth beat in the top strip, the third and seventh beats in the middle strip, and the fifth beat in the bottom strip). The cycles of the captured beats represent a rate of 62/min, indicating that at that sinus rate we could expect 1:1 conduction with mere first-degree block (compare with Figure 221).

This may still be hard to grasp, so turn your attention to the stalactitic arrows in the second strip. The first arrow indicates a P wave that represents a conducted sinus impulse; notice its distance from the preceding QRS complex (R-P interval). The second arrow points to the next P wave, whose impulse is not conducted (because its R-P interval is too short). The third arrow indicates the point at which the next P wave would have had to land to have an R-P interval equal to that of the conducted beat and presumably to again permit conduction.

The lessons to be learned from tracings like this are that an increased atrial rate is a handicap to A-V conduction because the faster the rate, the shorter the R-P interval after a conducted beat and that by looking at the cycle of captured beats, one can recognize the atrial rate at which 1:1 conduction would be possible and so obtain a better feel for the seriousness or mildness of the prevailing A-V conduction impairment.

For further application of these principles, see Figures 197, 221 and 224. Turn to each of them now and determine the atrial rate that should provide 1:1 conduction.

216

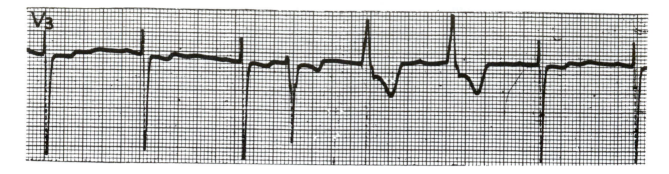

216

Diagnosis. **Sinus bradycardia** (rate 58/min) interrupted by a **VPB;** the next two sinus beats are conducted with RBBB **aberration** and with prolonged P-R intervals because of **concealed retrograde conduction** into the junction from the VPB (see laddergram).

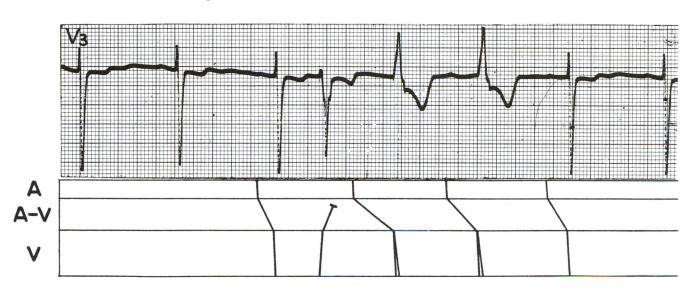

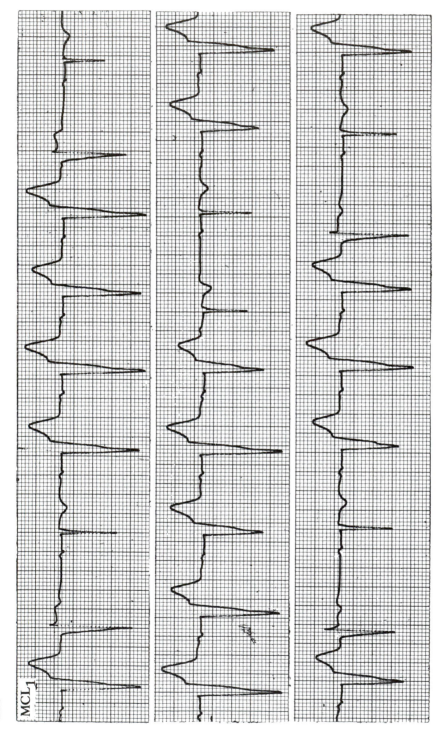

217

MCL₁

217

Diagnosis. Sinus rhythm with first-degree A-V block and **rate-dependent LBBB;** several **VPBs** followed by normal intraventricular conduction at the end of the longer postectopic cycles. The sixth beat in the second strip is an **APB** with **supernormal intraventricular conduction.** The cycle after the APB is also longer than the basic sinus cycle because of overdrive suppression of the sinus node by the APB and is therefore also normally conducted.

Special Points. One recognizes that the LBBB is rate-related by the fact that the postextrasystolic beats, ending somewhat longer cycles, are normally conducted.

Because the APB in the second strip is normally conducted despite the fact that it ends a shorter cycle than the cycles that end with LBBB (i.e., conduction is better than expected, better earlier than later), the intraventricular conduction qualifies as supernormal conduction.

218

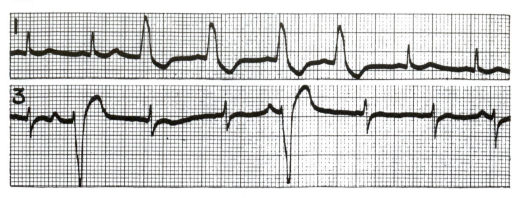

218

Diagnosis. **Sinus rhythm interrupted by APBs** that are conducted with **LBBB aberration.** In lead 1, the aberration persists in the next three conducted beats, the third of which may be another APB.

Special Point. This is another example of "critical rate," but with an extra wrinkle. In lead 1, the aberration develops with the shortening of the ventricular cycle, and it ceases when the cycle sufficiently lengthens. But if the second and last beats—ending cycles of 68 and 70—can be conducted normally, why cannot the fifth beat, which ends a longer cycle (72)?

The reason for this is that the second and last beats end cycles that began with normally conducted beats, whereas the fifth beat ends a cycle that began with a beat with LBBB. And when a cycle begins with BBB, the cycle, so far as the crucial bundle branch is concerned, is not appropriately measured from the beginning of QRS to the beginning of the next QRS. When a beat manifests BBB, the bundle branch involved is not activated until the contralateral impulse has had time to penetrate the septum and reach the initially blocked region (impulse 2 in figure), and this usually takes about 0.06 sec. Therefore, as far as the involved bundle branch is concerned, its cycle begins about halfway through the widened QRS complex. If one measures the cycle that ends with beat five beginning halfway through the QRS of beat four, one finds that it is actually shorter (66) than the cycles ending with the second and last beats (68 and 70).

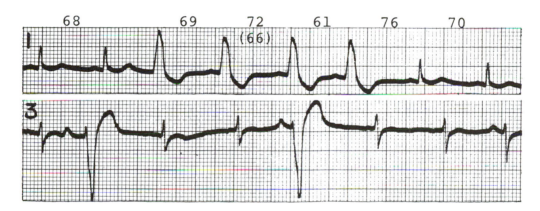

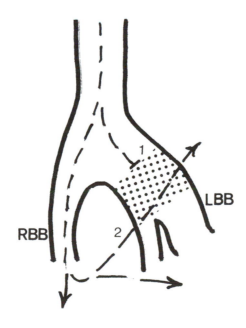

219

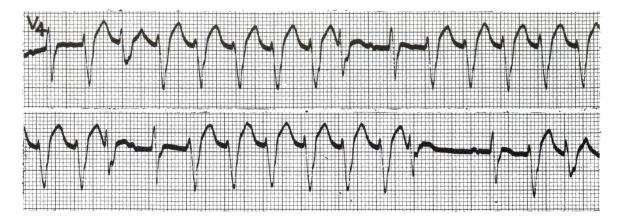

220

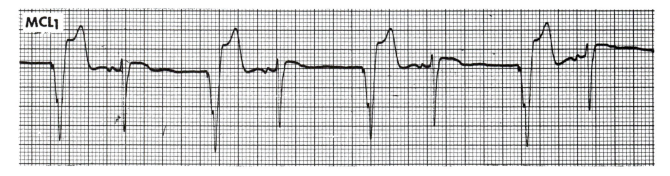

219

Diagnosis. **Sinus rhythm with first-degree A-V block,** repeated paroxysms of **ventricular tachycardia;** each paroxysm is terminated by a **VPB** from a presumably nearby focus.

Special Points. "Presumably" is used because the morphology of the terminating QRS complex is somewhat similar to the morphology of the preceding beats of the tachycardia; therefore, we can only say "presumably" because we know from experience that totally dissimilar beats can look remarkably alike in one lead.

Sinus P waves appear to march through the ventricular tachycardia at a rate of about 100/min.

The fact that the tachycardia is terminated by premature stimulus strongly suggests that it is reentrant and that the premature impulse has found the nonrefractory gap between the head and tail of the circulating wave.

220

Diagnosis. **Right ventricular demand pacemaker** with delayed retrograde conduction and **reciprocal beating** (see laddergram).

Special Points. The R-P interval of retrograde conduction after ectopic ventricular beats can be quite long (here, the R-P interval = 0.58 sec).

Note that, as usual, when a retrograde P wave is diphasic in V_1 or MCL_1, it is first negative and then positive, in contrast with the diphasic sinus P, which is usually positive and then negative, as in Figures 164 and 166.

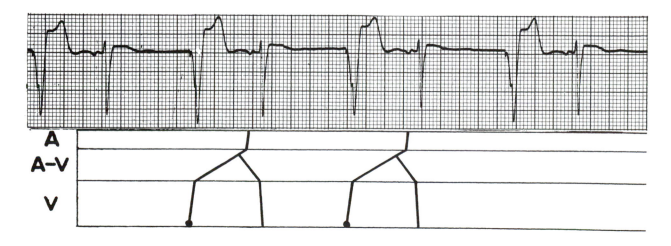

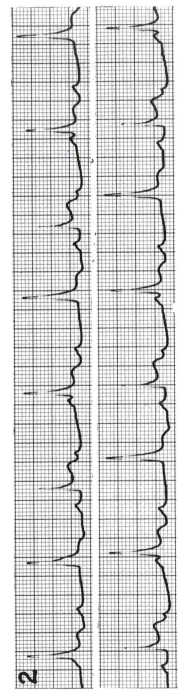

221

2

221

Diagnosis. A mild degree of A-V block combined with an **accelerated junctional rhythm** producing **A-V dissociation** with frequent **ventricular captures** (see laddergram); the capture beats have prolonged P-R intervals (0.26 sec). The morphology of the junctional beats, slightly different from that of the conducted ones, is presumably due to Type B aberration—see discussion of Figures 150 and 164. (Tracing from a patient with an acute inferior infarction.)

Special Points. This tracing, like Figures 150 and 164, illustrates some important blind spots and little appreciated clues. Such tracings are often classified as high-grade block because so few of the sinus impulses are conducted—here, only 5 of 26. But that is not the way to assess the severity of incomplete A-V block. Instead of dwelling on the beats that are not conducted, one should concentrate on those that are, because obviously they indicate what is required for conduction. If one observes the characteristics of the capture beats, one soon sees that conduction occurs only when the R-P interval reaches 0.56 sec, and then it occurs with some prolongation of the P-R. If this R-P is added to the P-R, the sum equals the cycle ending with a capture beat, and that cycle length represents the atrial rate, that is, 76/min, at which one could expect 1:1 A-V conduction. Obviously, anyone whose A-V junction is capable of conducting every atrial beat—with a little P-R prolongation—at a rate of 76/min has only minor A-V block.

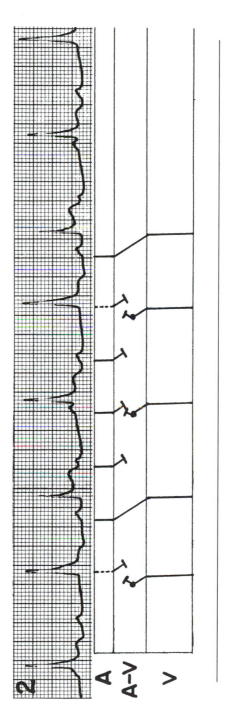

222

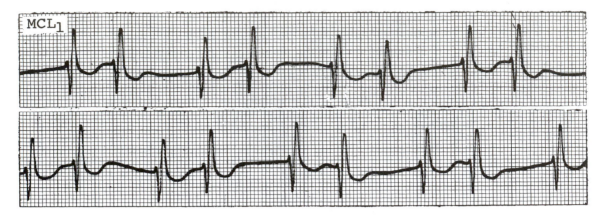

223

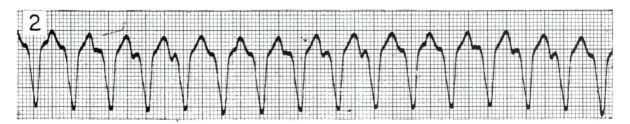

222

Diagnosis. **Junctional tachycardia** (rate 130/min) with **3 : 2 Wenckebach** conduction below the junctional pacemaker and **RBBB.** (From a patient with fatal digitalis intoxication.)

Special Points. The rSR′ pattern is so characteristic of RBBB that one must assume that the rhythm is supraventricular. Because the beats are grouped in pairs, one immediately thinks of 3 : 2 Wenckebach periods, and the smoothly sagging ST segments are eloquent of digitalis effect. There are no P waves, so the atria are silent (or possibly depolarized retrogradely during each QRS complex).

Putting all these points together, the above diagnosis is logically arrived at (see laddergram).

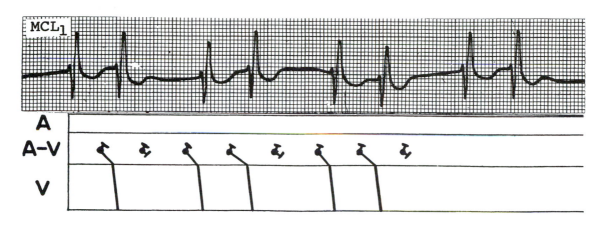

223

Diagnosis. **Ventricular tachycardia** (rate 150/min) with 5 : 4 **retrograde (V-A) Wenckebachs**—see laddergram.

Special Point. Retrograde conduction to the atria occurs in nearly half of ventricular tachycardias.

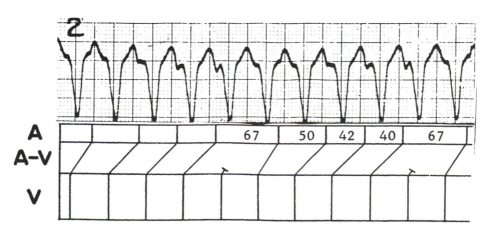

224

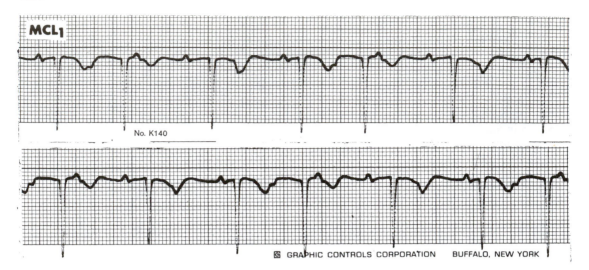

MCL₁

No. K140

Ⓖ GRAPHIC CONTROLS CORPORATION   BUFFALO, NEW YORK

224

Diagnosis. **Sinus tachycardia** (rate 110/min) with **Type I A-V block** manifested as 3 : 2 Wenckebachs alternating with 2 : 1 conduction (see laddergram).

Special Point. The cycles of the captured beats (0.66–0.70 sec) inform us that if only the patient had a somewhat more modest atrial rate of about 90/min—instead of the conduction-inhibiting tachycardia—he would be able to conduct every atrial impulse. Yet tracings such as this are often mistakenly overdiagnosed as "high-grade" or "advanced" A-V block because the majority of the impulses are not conducted (as though that were entirely due to the A-V block). Compare Figures 150, 164, 170, 197, 215, and 221.

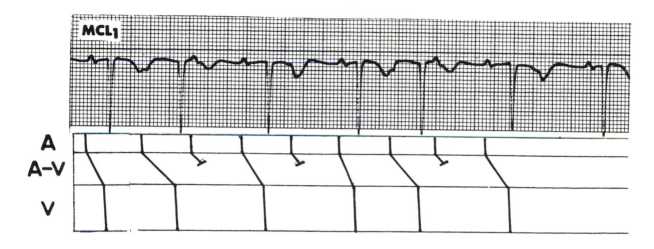

225

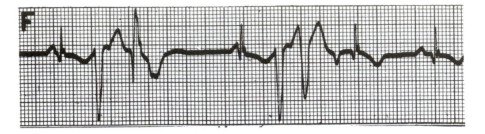

226

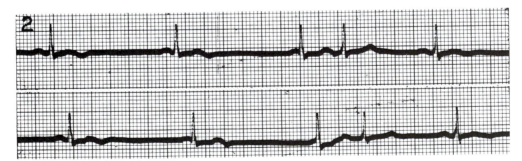

225

Diagnosis. The basic rhythm cannot be satisfactorily determined from this short strip. Taking it beat by beat and assuming that the last beat is a conducted sinus beat, then the first beat is a dissociated beat (sinus from junctional) with a pair of bifocal **ventricular extrasystoles** with retrograde conduction, the R-P interval of the second being longer than that of the first. A similar sequence follows: a dissociated beat followed by a pair of ventricular extrasystoles. Because the interval between the second pair of ectopic beats is shorter than that between the previous pair, the second R-P interval is even more prolonged and therefore a **reciprocal beat** results (see laddergram).

Special Point. This tracing reemphasizes the facility for retrograde conduction to the atria, the potential for retrograde Wenckebach conduction, and the fact that delayed conduction favors reentry.

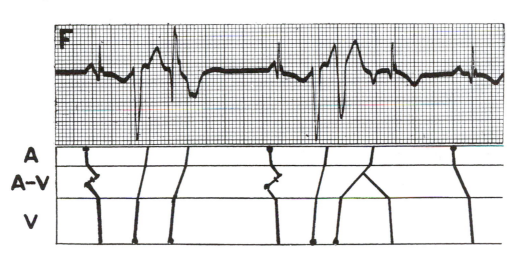

226

Diagnosis. **Atrial bigeminy** (mostly nonconducted) with resulting **junctional escape** (see laddergram).

Special Point. Another victim of overdiagnosis. This patient was diagnosed as having a "funny sort of block" and had a temporary pacemaker inserted—for APBs!

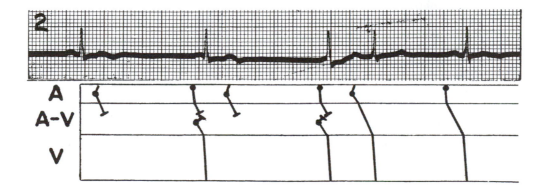

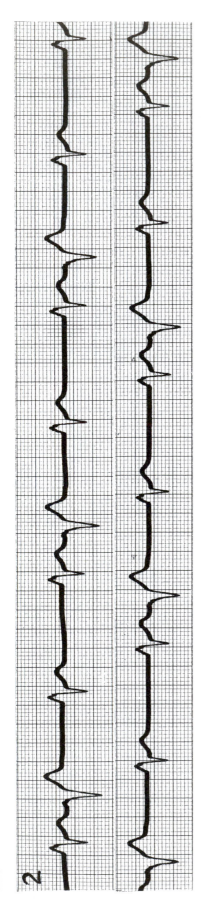

227

2

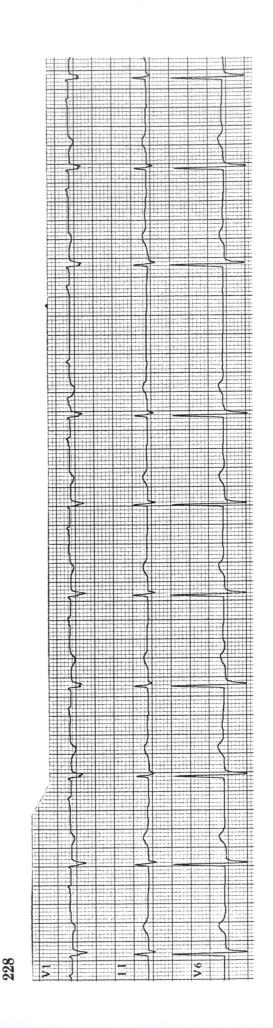

228

V1

11

V6

227

Diagnosis. **Atrial standstill** (?sinus arrest) with idioventricular rhythm (rate 48/min) interrupted by VPBs every third beat.

228

Diagnosis. Sinus rhythm with **first-degree A-V block** (PR = 0.27 sec) interrupted by a pair of **nonconducted APBs.**

Special Point. Failure of conduction of the second of the pair of APBs is probably due to concealed conduction of the first into the junction (see laddergram and compare with Figure 234).

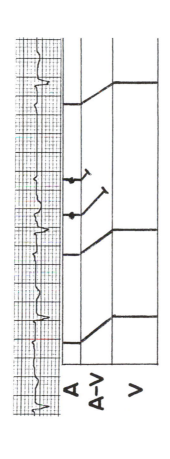

A
A–V
V

229

V1

II

V6

230

V1

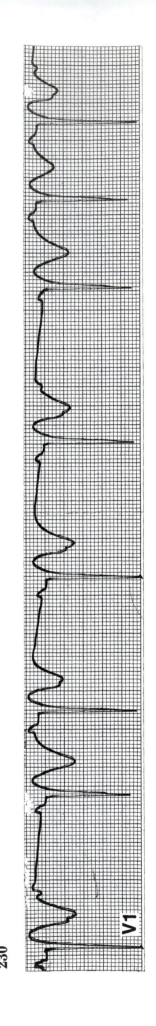

229

Diagnosis. Apparent complete A-V block is interrupted by a single **supernormally conducted (captured) beat**; **idiojunctional rhythm with RBBB** and **left anterior hemiblock.**

Special Point. When impaired conduction is interrupted by surprisingly good conduction, it is called "supernormal"; in fact, it is not better than normal, rather it is better **than expected,** that is, better earlier in the cycle than later. In this case the conducted beat enables us to recognize the mechanism of the independent rhythm as junctional because the conducted beat has a shape identical with that of the independent beats (compare Figures 210 and 254).

230

Diagnosis. Sinus rhythm interrupted by frequent **nonconducted APBs,** singly and in pairs (arrows); one junctional escape beat (E).

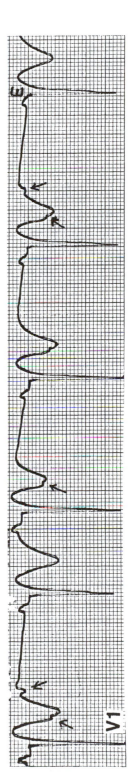

V1

231

V1

II

V6

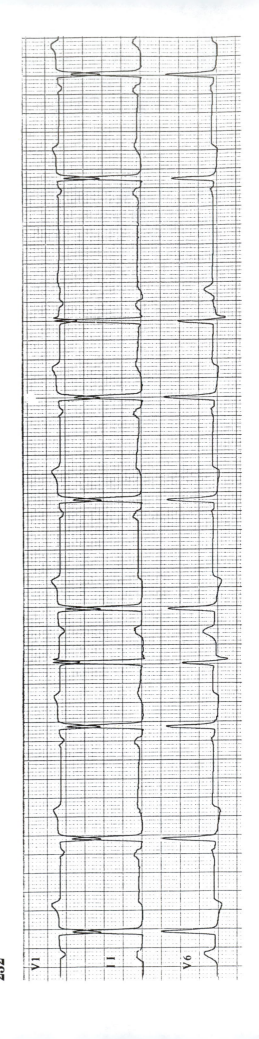

232

V1

II

V6

231

Diagnosis. **Atrial tachycardia** (rate 133/min) with **varying A-V conduction.**

232

Diagnosis. **Sinus bradycardia** interrupted by **two junctional premature beats** with different coupling intervals and with minor **ventricular aberration,** the first interpolated, the second followed by a fully compensatory pause.

Special Point. Note that the interpolated beat lengthens the P-R interval of the next sinus beat because it has left the junction somewhat refractory and therefore delayed the next descending impulse. Both junctional prematures manifest mild aberration due to incipient RBBB (secondary r wave in V_1 and shrinkage of negative deflection, with less tall R in V_6 and development of S wave).

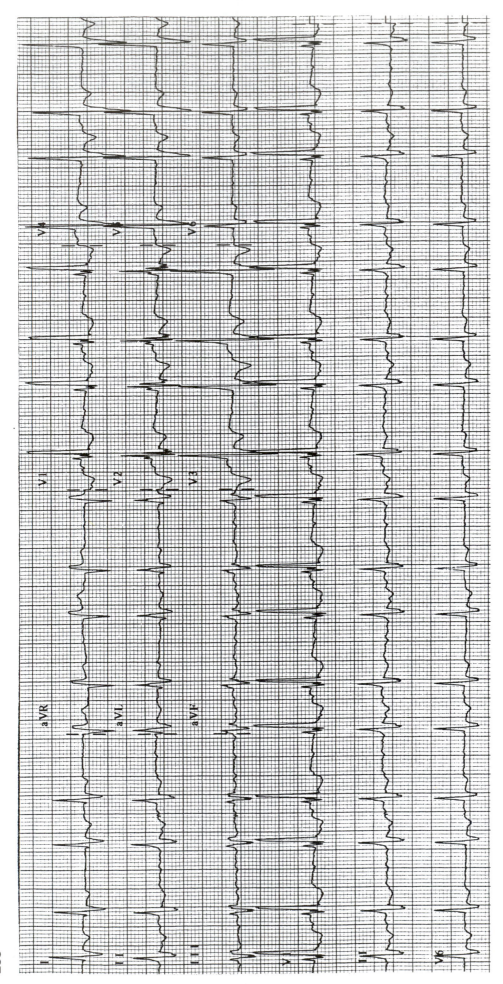

233

Diagnosis. Atrial flutter (rate 300/min) with alternating **2 : 1 and 4 : 1 conduction, RBBB** with possible right ventricular hypertrophy.

Special Point. Whenever 2 : 1 and 4 : 1 conduction alternate in atrial flutter, it is due to 2 : 1 "filtering" at a higher level in the junction with a 3 : 2 Wenckebach developing at a lower level (compare Figures 126, 270, and 275).

Here, the flutter waves are unusually inconspicuous but are clearly discernible in the inferior leads 2, 3 and aVF. (The primary T-wave changes, especially seen in lead 1 and V leads, are probably due to anterior ischemia; and the R´ of 16 mm in V_1 suggests right ventricular hypertrophy).

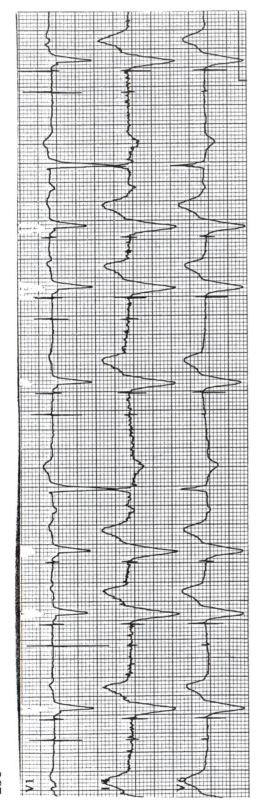

234

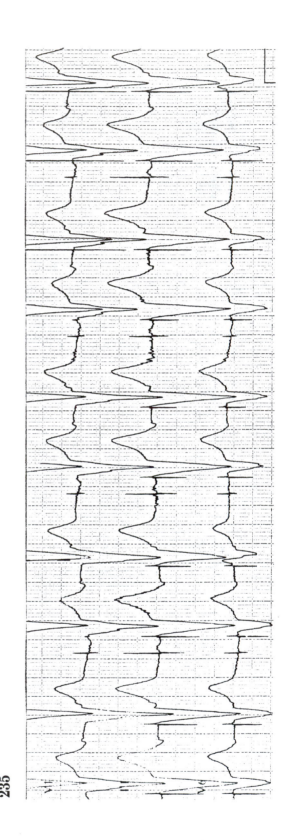

235

234

Diagnosis. Dual-chambered pacemaker in both sequential and atrial-tracking modes; APBs with prolonged P-to-R intervals and **reciprocal beats.**

Special Point. In a dual-chambered pacemaker tracing, a single spike identifies atrial tracking. But why are only the atrial-tracked beats followed by retrograde conduction to the atria? Presumably, it is because of the longer P-R interval of the tracked APB that favors reentry and therefore reciprocal beating. The P" waves of the APBs are best seen in V_1; the retrograde P waves are well seen in all three leads.

235

Diagnosis. Dual-chambered pacemaker in both sequential and atrial-tracking modes.

Special Point. Throughout the strip, sequential and atrial-tracking modes alternate; the sequentially paced beats are conducted retrogradely to the atria, the retrograde P waves are tracked, and a form of bigeminy results.

236

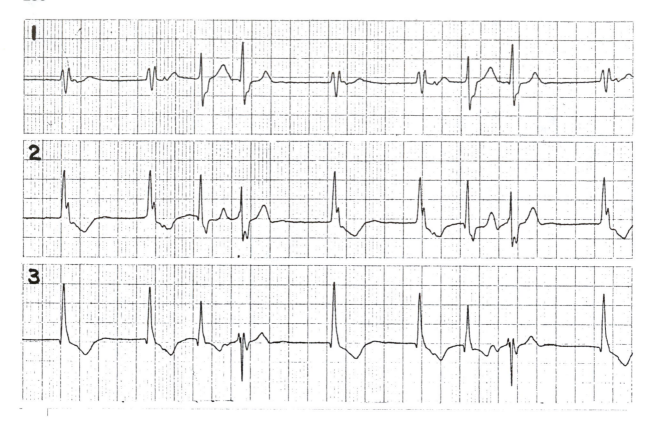

236

Diagnosis. Accelerated idioventricular rhythm with progressive delay in retrograde conduction producing a **reciprocating rhythm** for two beats; the first of the two reciprocal beats is conducted with **RBBB** and the second with **left anterior hemiblock** as well.

Special Point. When a sequence of dissimilar beats recurs, it is sometimes called an allorhythmia.

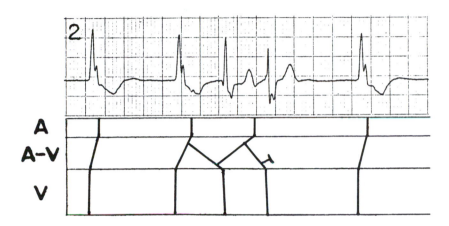

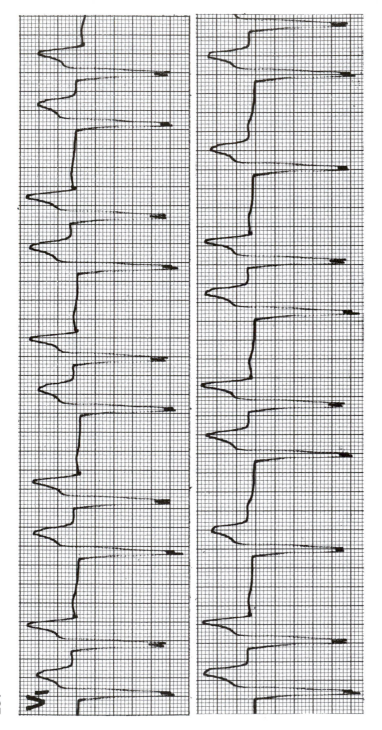

237

Diagnosis. **Right ventricular tachycardia** with 3 : 2 and 2 : 1 **exit block** out of the ectopic focus and with retrograde conduction to the atria (arrows).

Special Point. Note the longer R-P interval after the second of each pair of beats. The developing retrograde Wenckebach is aborted by the dropped beat of the 3 : 2 Wenckebach out of the ectopic ventricular focus (in laddergram, e = ectopic focus in ventricle).

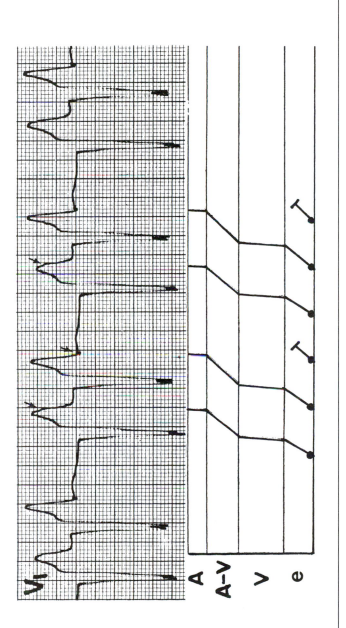

238

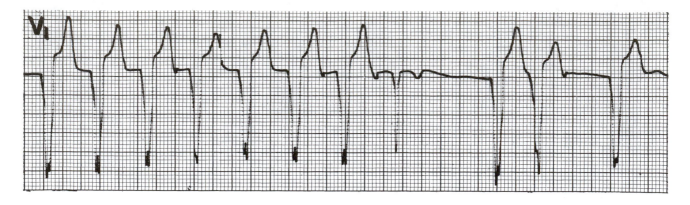

238

Diagnosis. **This tracing is from the same patient as in Figure 177. Right ventricular tachycardia** with **retrograde conduction** to atria with progressive lengthening of R-P intervals (arrows); the paroxysm of tachycardia ceases in the middle of the strip at the same time that critical lengthening of the R-P interval results in a **reciprocal beat** (ventricular "echo," see laddergram). The returning ventricular beat is followed by a **VPB** with retrograde conduction.

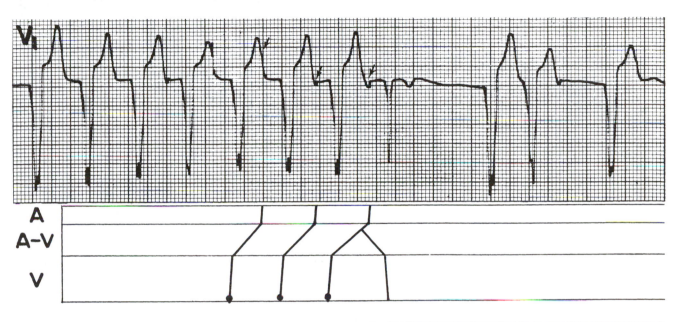

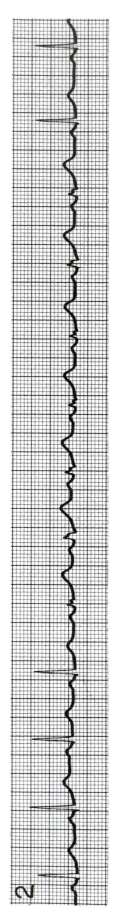

2

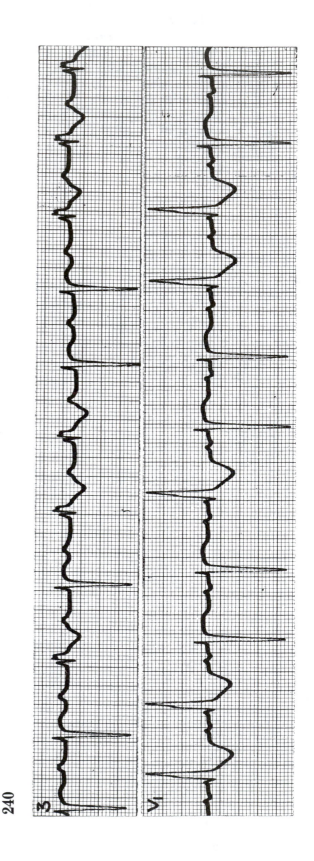

3

V₁

239

Diagnosis. Sinus rhythm with rate-dependent LBBB.

Special Point. Note that at the beginning of the strip, normal I-V conduction prevails, with the cycle as short as 0.72 sec; on the other hand, after the LBBB has developed, it persists even

though the cycle lengthens beyond 0.72 sec, and normal conduction resumes only when the ventricular cycle reaches 0.78 sec. (For a detailed explanation, see Figure 218.)

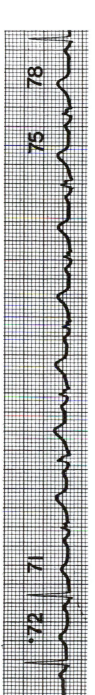

240

Diagnosis. Sinus rhythm with potential Type I A-V block and **intermittent RBBB** (unrelated to rate).

Special Points. Because the P-R intervals differ between leads 3 and V_1 and are reciprocally related to the associated R-P interval (the shorter R-P is associated with a longer P-R in lead 3, whereas a longer R-P is associated with a shorter

P-R in V_1) there is cogent evidence of Type I A-V block.

Of course, faster paper speeds and photographic recordings might reveal subtle differences in the R-R intervals, accounting for the intermittent development of RBBB, but from this routine clinical tracing, it is impossible to relate the development of RBBB to cycle length.

241

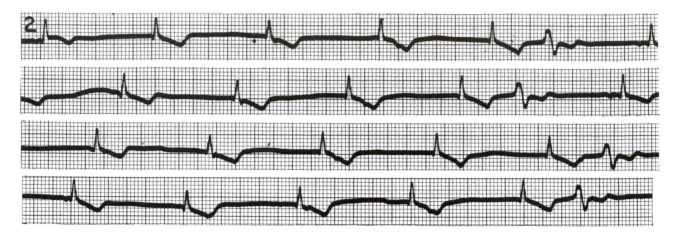

242

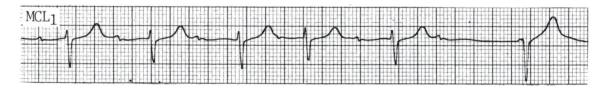

241

Diagnosis. **A-V dissociation** between two junctional pacemakers, with **ventricular captures** by the higher pacemaker occurring every sixth or seventh beat; the capture beats are **aberrantly conducted** (upper laddergram).

Special Point. In this case, the P-P intervals are constant, and this establishes the diagnosis of two independent junctional pacemakers rather than junctional rhythm with reciprocal beating (lower laddergram and see Figure 112).

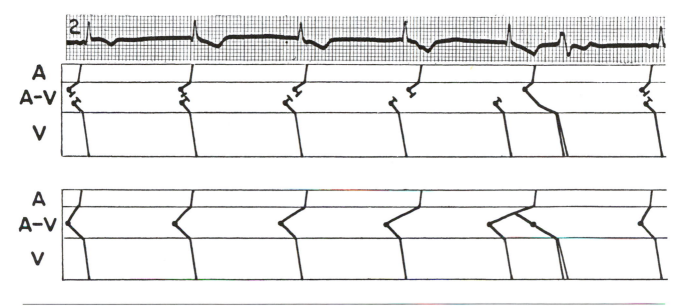

242

Diagnosis. The first three beats show classic Wenckebach behavior, but then, after further shortening of the R-P interval, the P-R interval paradoxically also shortens. This better than expected conduction immediately makes one think of supernormal conduction. However, (a) supernormal conduction is a refuge of the diagnostically destitute, and (b) genuine supernormal A-V conduction almost always occurs after a retro-

gradely conducted impulse in the A-V junction. Therefore, another explanation is needed.

Conduction delay favors reentry, and it may well be that the third P-R interval represents the degree of delay necessary for reentry to occur. If so, the apparently shortened P-R interval may not represent conduction at all but may be the result of reentry in the A-V junction (see laddergram).

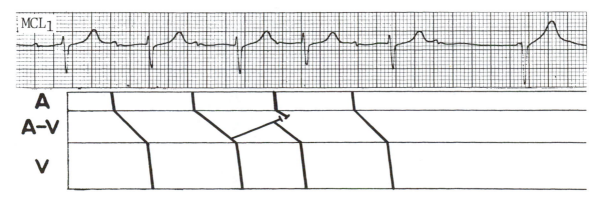

243

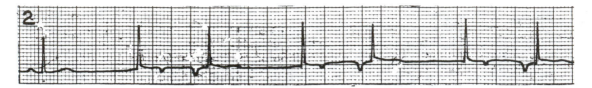

244

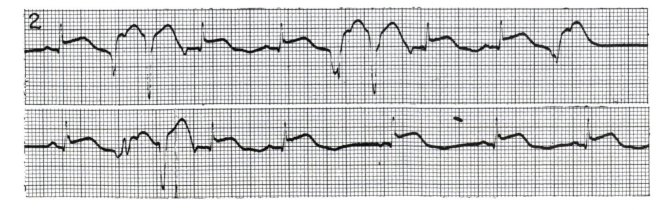

243

Diagnosis. **After the initial sinus beat, the ensuing pause ends with junctional escape,** which initiates reentry in the A-V junction. A plausible explanation for the ensuing relationships is shown in the first laddergram. The reciprocating impulse succeeds in reaching the atria twice but is blocked anterogradely and fails to reach the ventricles.

The second laddergram depicts another possibility: that the retrograde impulse reaches the atria twice, first via a fast pathway and then via a slow pathway; reentry results from the slower retrograde conduction and produces a **reciprocal beat** (ventricular echo).

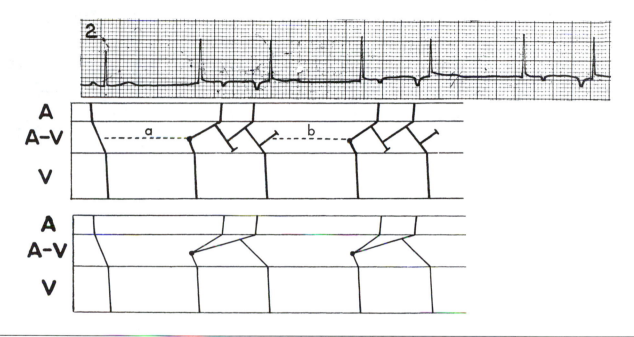

244

Diagnosis. **Sinus rhythm with single and paired bifocal VPBs and retrograde conduction** to atria. The R-P interval of the second of each pair is longer than the first; this favors reentry, and a **reciprocal beat** (ventricular echo) results. The sixth beat in the bottom strip is a **junctional** (or atrial) **escape** ending a **sinus pause.** (The conducted beats show the current of injury of acute inferior infarction.)

245

MCL₁

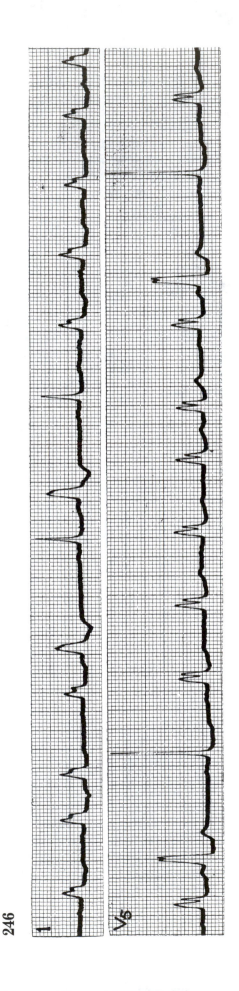

246

1

V₅

245

Diagnosis. Double tachycardia: ventricular tachycardia (rate 130/min) dissociated from **atrial** (?sinus) **tachycardia** (rate 126/min). The apparent changing peaks of the ventricular complex are due to the deeply negative P waves marching through them. The 7th beat in the top strip and the 2nd and 11th beats in the bottom strip are **VPBs.** The last beat in the top strip and the third in the bottom strip are **ventricular captures;** the next to last beat in the top strip and the fourth beat in the bottom strip are definite **fusion beats.**

246

Diagnosis. Sinus rhythm with intra-atrial block and **rate-dependent LBBB;** four **VPBs** and three **APBs.**

Special Points. Note that the VPBs have an LBBB pattern, but this does not identify their origin. Although this pattern is typical of right ventricular ectopy, it is also sometimes seen as part of the "concordant positivity" pattern of left ventricular ectopy (see Figure 70).

The LBBB is recognized as rate dependent by the fact that the longest cycles (after each VPB) all end with a QRS complex that is more normally conducted. The absent septal q wave in these left-sided leads (1 and V$_5$) is undoubtedly an early indication of LBBB.

The third and last beats in lead 1 and the eighth beat in V$_5$ are APBs; note the slight deformity of preceding T waves due to superimposition of premature P' waves.

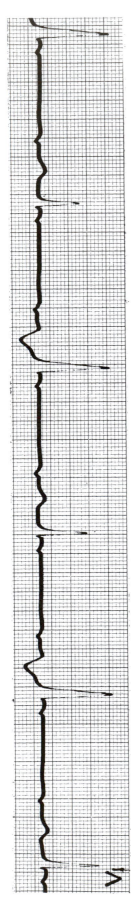

247

V₁

247

Diagnosis. Sinus rhythm with 2 : 1 A-V block and alternating LBBB.

Special Points. In this example of 2 : 1 A-V block, it is impossible to say whether it is more likely Type I or Type II. A prolonged P-R interval and no BBB would strongly favor Type I, whereas a normal P-R interval and a BBB would favor Type II but not exclude Type I.

The most plausible explanation for the alternating LBBB is simultaneous 4 : 1 LBBB with 2 : 1 RBBB (see diagram).

Key: HB = bundle of His; R = right bundle branch; L = left bundle branch; LBBB = left bundle-branch block; AVB = no A-V conduction; NL = normal intraventricular conduction.

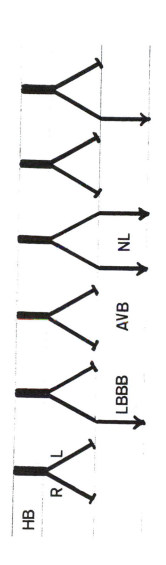

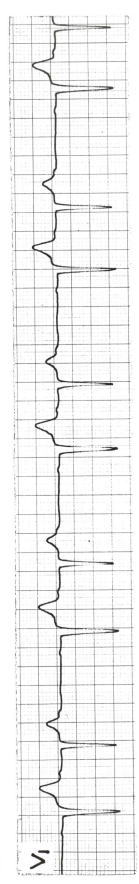

248

V₁

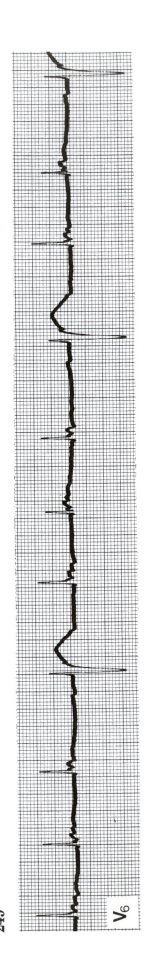

249

V₆

248

Diagnosis. Sinus rhythm with 3 : 2 A-V Wenckebach periods; paradoxical critical rate phenomenon in left bundle branch.

Special Point. Each pair of QRS complexes manifests a degree of LBBB greater in the first QRS than in the second. When conduction is better at the end of a shorter cycle than at the end of a longer one, there are many explanatory theories, for example, supernormal conduction of the early beats or vagal effect on the later beat. Probably the most acceptable theory is that it represents a phase 4 phenomenon (see Figure 157).

Another possibility is that the first beat of each pair is not conducted but represents junctional escape with what is sometimes called Type B aberration, that is, abnormal conduction through the ventricles because of abnormal conduction above the ventricles (see Figure 150).

A third possibility is that the first beat in each pair is a ventricular escape beat.

Note: We should never be surprised when the more complex arrhythmias defy us with more than one equally plausible interpretation. Remember Rosenbaum's dictum: "After all, every self-respecting arrhythmia has at least three possible interpretations."

249

Diagnosis. Sinus rhythm with 4 : 3 and 3 : 2 A-V Wenckebach periods. The long cycles of the dropped beats end with **ventricular escape.**

Special Points. The P-R intervals are unusually long (up to 0.74 sec), although they can be much longer and have been reported as long as over 1.00 sec, and there is paradoxical lengthening of the last cycle before the dropped beat—something that happens in a significant minority of Wenckebachs. In the classic Wenckebach period, the R-R interval becomes progressively

shorter because the P-R increments progressively decrease. In a significant minority, however, the P-R increment of the last conducted beat before the blocked beat paradoxically increases, and this correspondingly lengthens the R-R interval.

The presumed escape beats could, of course, be conducted with an unexpected paradoxical aberration (RBBB with anterior hemiblock), but this morphology of the QRS complex in V_6 makes an ectopic ventricular mechanism much more likely.

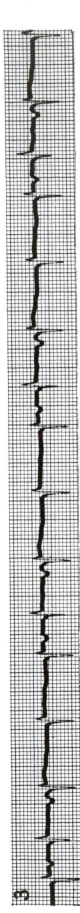

250

3

250

Diagnosis. **Accelerated junctional rhythm** (rate 85/min) with progressive delay in retrograde conduction and **reciprocal beating** (see laddergram).

Special Point. The differential diagnosis is of course dissociation between two junctional pacemakers, one controlling the atria and the other the ventricles, with occasional capture of the ventricles by the higher junctional pacemaker (see Figure 181). Differentiating features here are that the P waves are irregular, and they bear a recurring relationship to the QRS complexes.

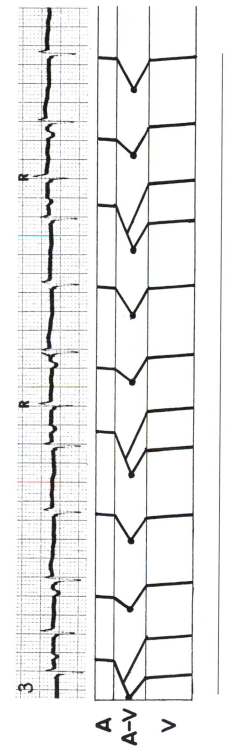

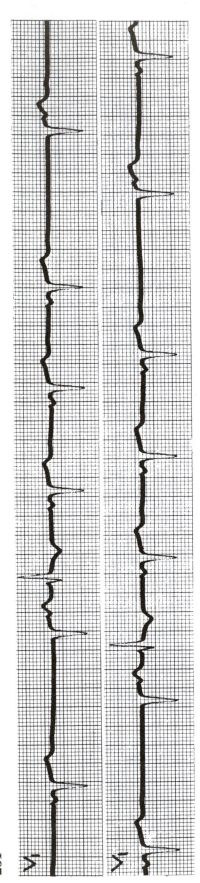

251

Diagnosis. Sinus rhythm with 5 : 4 Wenckebachs out of the sinus node; the long pause caused by the blocked sinus impulse ends with **junctional escape**, and the next sinus beat is conducted with **RBBB aberration.**

Special Point. The P-P intervals show the typical "footprints" of the Wenckebach, for example, in the top strip they measure consecutively 199, 114, 108, 105, and 196.

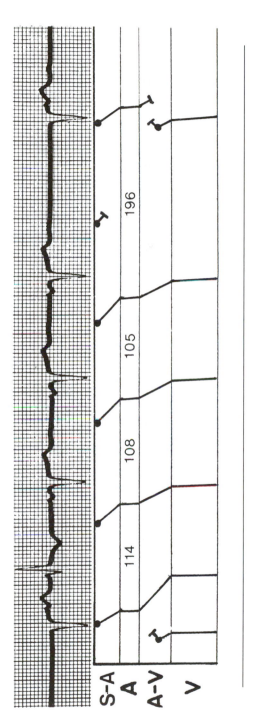

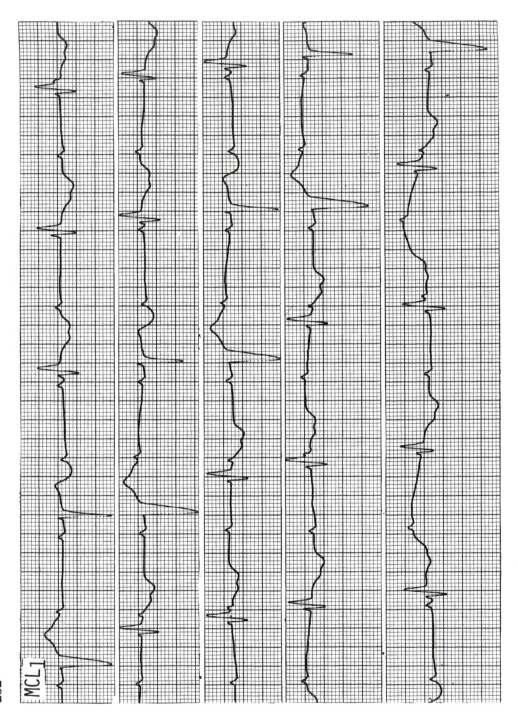

MCL₁

252

Diagnosis. Sinus rhythm with 2 : 1 A-V block and **LBBB; ventricular escape** at a rate (41/min) slightly faster than the conductible atrial rate; several **fusion beats** result (second beat in top strip, third in second strip, fourth in third strip, and fifth in fourth strip).

Special Points. Although the idioventricular beats have an rSR″ pattern, strongly suggesting a supraventricular origin with RBBB, they

are more likely an exceptional form of left ventricular ectopy; when they fuse with conducted LBBB beats, the QRS pattern narrows and normalizes, indicating simultaneous activation of the two ventricles.

Furthermore, if the sinus beats that are conducted are conducted with *left* BBB, it is highly unlikely that junctional beats would be conducted with *right* BBB.

253

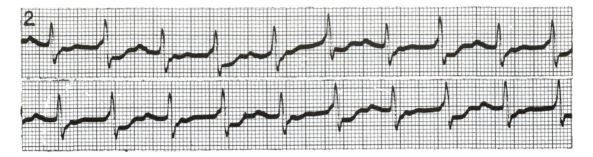

254

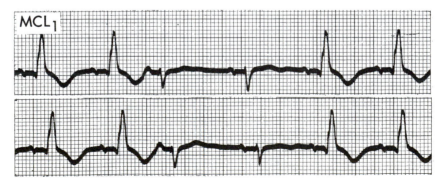

253

Diagnosis. **Sinus tachycardia** (rate 152/min) with recurrent 3 : 2 **A-V Wenckebach** periods and frequent **APBs.**

Special Point. At first glance, it looks as though the ventricular rhythm is regular, but if measured carefully, the QRS cycles alternate. The resulting pairing of the beats suggests 3 : 2 conduction, and the Wenckebach pattern immediately becomes suspect. Careful measurement of the P-P intervals, however, reveals that every third P wave is slightly early, so the pairing is due to a combination of the 3 : 2 conduction plus the prematurity of every third P wave (see laddergram).

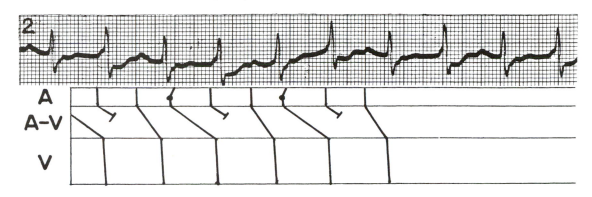

254

Diagnosis. **Sinus rhythm with RBBB; APBs** with normalized ventricular complexes (and in the beats ending the postectopic cycles).

Special Point. Whenever earlier conduction is better than later, that is, better than expected, one may invoke supernormal conduction (compare Figures 159, 163, and 166). "Overdrive suppression" by the APB is what makes the next cycle long enough for normal conduction to again occur.

255

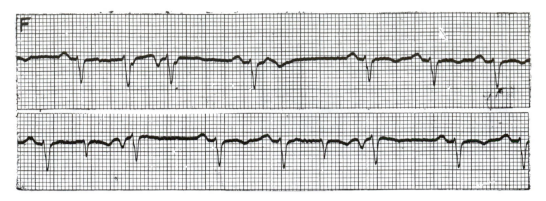

255

Diagnosis. **Sinus rhythm interrupted by APBs** with **first-degree A-V block;** consequent **reciprocal beats** (see laddergram).

Special Point. The prolonged P-R interval of the APB favors reentry (see similar situation interrupting the A-V Wenckebach phenomenon in Figure 182).

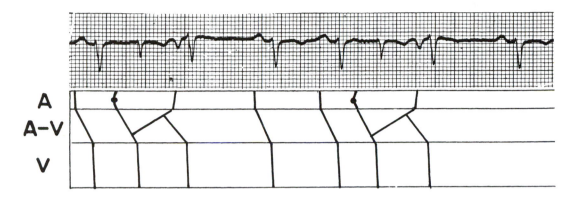

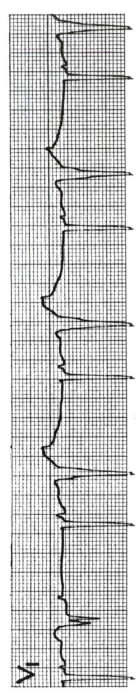

256

256

Diagnosis. **Junctional rhythm with ventricular bigeminy; retrograde conduction** to the atria after each beat (see laddergram).

Special Point. Note that the R-P interval differs as between the junctional and the ectopic ventricular beat. This is because retrograde con-

duction with junctional rhythm equals the difference between anterograde and retrograde conduction, whereas with the ectopic ventricular beat, the R-P interval is a true measure of retrograde conduction per se (see laddergram and Figure 103).

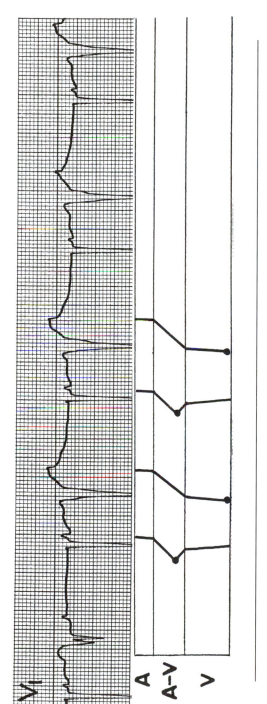

257

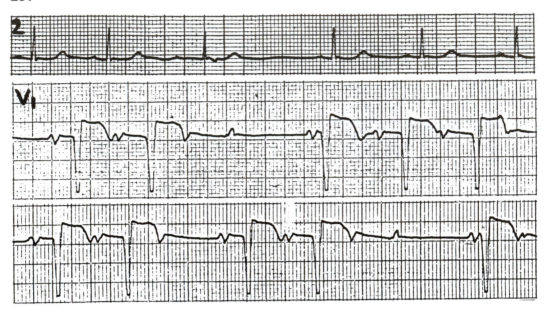

257

Diagnosis. **Top strip (lead 2): there is a
developing A-V Wenckebach period that is
aborted, when the P-R reaches a critical
length, by an atrial echo** (reversed reciprocal
beat). The bottom two strips (lead V_1) contain
completed **3 : 2 Wenckebach periods.** On two oc-
casions, the sinus impulse that fails to reach the
ventricles nevertheless returns to the atria as an
atrial echo (see laddergram).

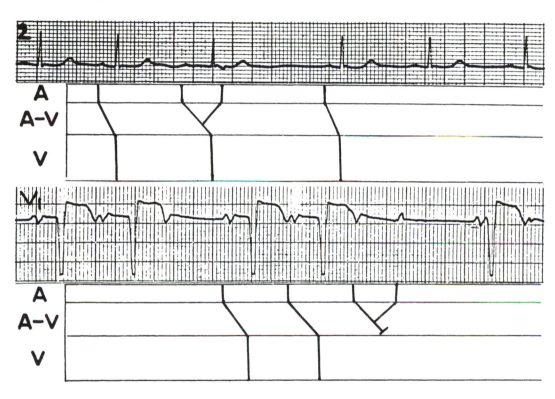

258

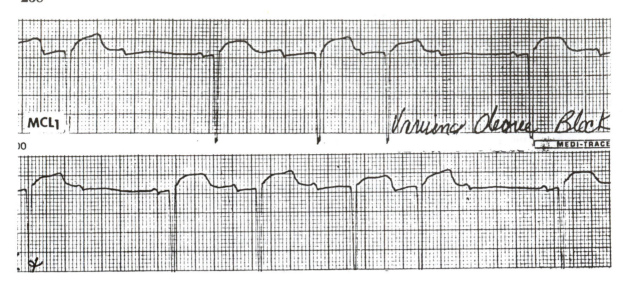

MCL₁

259

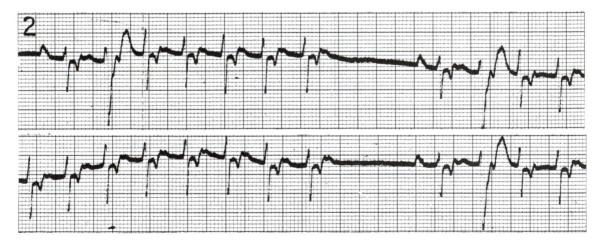

258

Diagnosis. In both strips of this continuous tracing, a developing A-V Wenckebach is unexpectedly interrupted by a shortening of the P-R interval, despite associated shortening of the R-P interval. This might be explained by supernormal conduction, but it is more likely that critical lengthening of the P-R has opened the door to reentry and that consequent **reciprocation** in the A-V junction (see laddergram) explains the sudden abrogation of the usual R-P/P-R reciprocity (compare Figures 182 and 195).

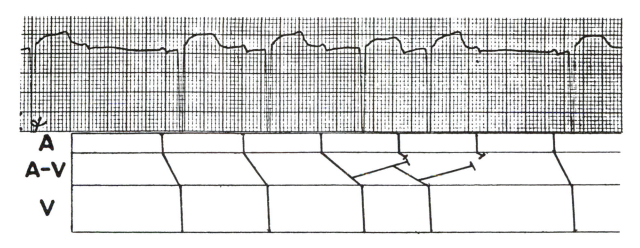

259

Diagnosis. The prolonged P-R intervals (0.21– 0.24 sec) of the sinus beats favor the development of reentry, and orthodromic tachycardia is initiated. The second beat in each group develops **ventricular aberration,** the pattern of which suggests RBBB with left anterior hemiblock.

Special Point. This is a good example of delayed anterograde conduction favoring retrograde reentry which, in turn, produces an atrial echo and initiates a reciprocating tachycardia (see laddergram).

It also nicely illustrates the fact that the most likely beat to develop aberrant ventricular conduction is the second beat in a row because it is the only beat that ends a short cycle preceded by a relatively long cycle.

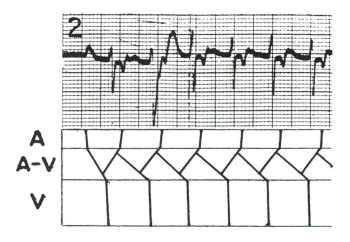

260

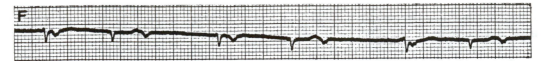

260

Diagnosis. **Junctional rhythm** with retrograde conduction to atria. In each pair of beats, the R-P interval is longer with the second than with the first; **concealed reentrant conduction** discharges the junctional pacemaker and produces a longer cycle (see laddergram).

Special Point. The long cycle is associated with a longer R-P interval, suggesting a causal relationship; when delayed conduction appears to be implicated, one should always suspect the operation of reentry.

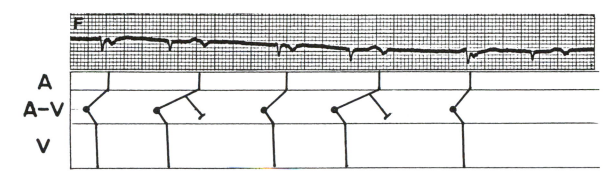

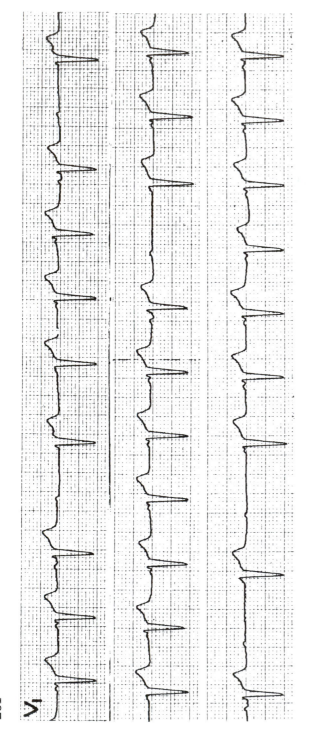

261

V₁

261

Diagnosis. Sinus rhythm with repeated Wenckebach periods.

Special Point. Note the "skipped" conduction. The P-R interval reaches 0.75 sec, and most of the conducted P-R intervals are longer than the R-R intervals. Compare with Figure 130.

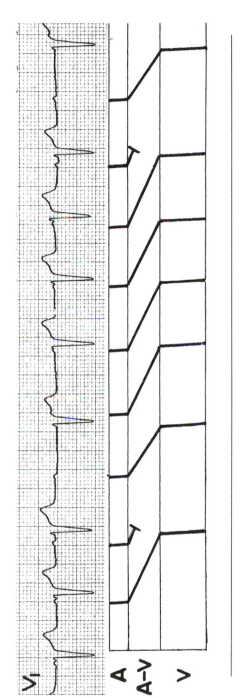

262

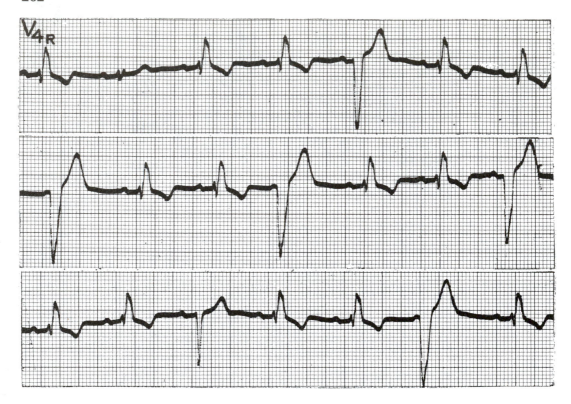

263

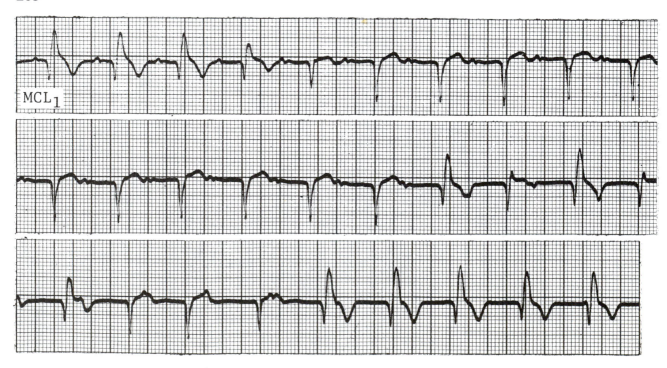

262

Diagnosis. **Sinus rhythm with RBBB; right ventricular parasystole; ventricular fusion beats.**

Special Point. Remember that when an ectopic focus is on the same side as a bundle-branch block, fusion beats are narrower than either of the component complexes and often look surprisingly normal (compare Figures 138 and 192). In this tracing, the fusion beats are the second and fifth beats in the top strip, the last beat in the second strip, and the third beat in the bottom strip. Note how normal the fusion complex looks in the bottom strip.

263

Diagnosis. **Sinus rhythm with first-degree A-V block** (P-R = 0.32–0.56 sec) competing with an **accelerated idioventricular rhythm** from the left ventricle; **ventricular fusion beats.** (The pattern of both conducted and ectopic complexes reveals the underlying anteroseptal infarction.)

Special Point. Because the P-R intervals of the conducted beats are inversely related to their R-P intervals, there is obviously a latent or potential second degree Type I A-V block.

264

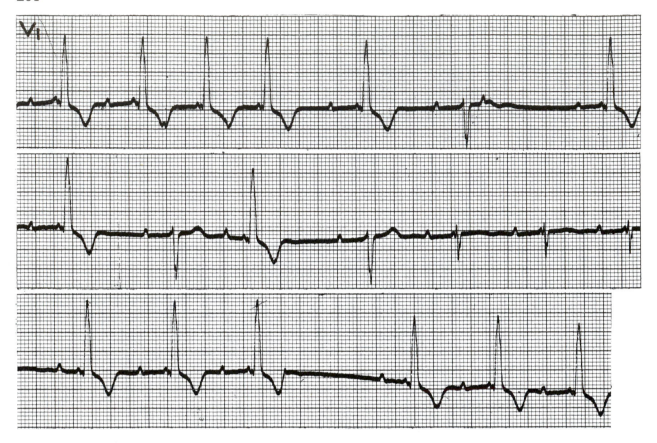

264

Diagnosis. **Sinus rhythm with Type I A-V block** and **rate-dependent RBBB; APBs.**

Special Points. First of all, the little blips at the beginning of each positive QRS complex are part of the QRS and not P waves. In the top strip, the third and fourth beats are APBs, and a non-conducted APB follows the sixth beat. Another nonconducted APB follows the third beat in the bottom strip.

There are three patterns of intraventricular conduction: RBBB, exemplified by the first five beats in the top strip; more or less normal con-duction (sixth beat in top strip, second and fourth beats in second strip); and an early stage of in-complete RBBB, as in the last three beats in the middle strip. (Note that the earliest sign of RBBB in V_1 is often a shrinkage of the S wave.) Notice that the full-blown RBBB pattern is found in the shortest cycles—64 to 103—(conventional aberra-tion) and longest cycles—147 to 164—(paradoxi-cal aberration, probably a phase 4 phenomenon; see Figure 157), whereas the more normal con-duction patterns are found at the end of interme-diate cycle lengths—88 to 129.

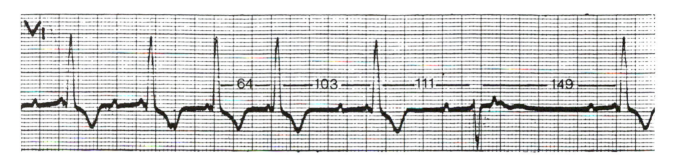

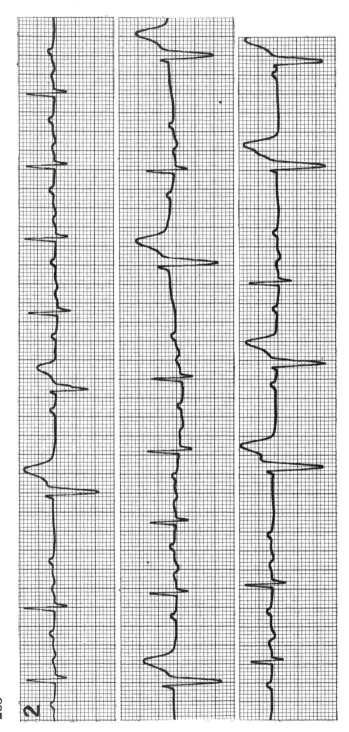

2

265

Diagnosis. Type II second-degree A-V block; ventricular escape and fusion beats. The ventricular escapes are probably **parasystolic,** in which case there must be **exit block** from the parasystolic focus.

Special Points. Despite the prolonged P-R interval and the absence of BBB, a combination characteristic of Type I block, this must be classified as Type II block because consecutive atrial impulses are conducted with unchanging P-R in-

tervals before the dropped beats. After each dropped beat, the lengthened cycle ends with one or two escaping ventricular parasystolic beats; the fourth beat in the top strip and the fourth beat in the bottom strip are fusion beats between a second parasystolic impulse and the sinus impulse. Exit block must be postulated because parasystolic beats do not always put in an appearance when expected (arrows).

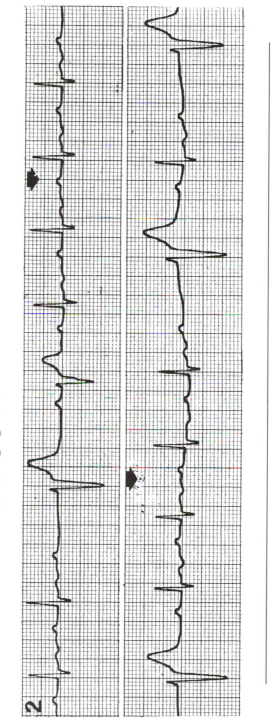

2

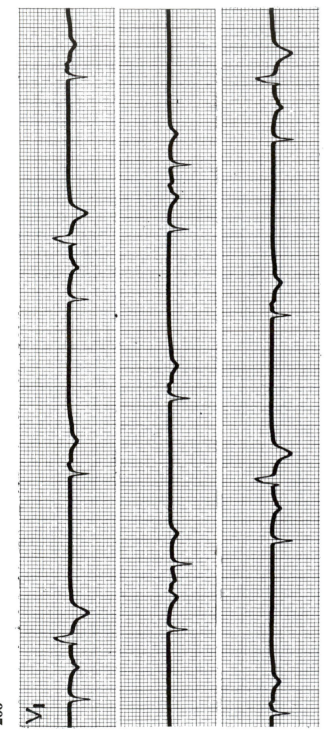

Diagnosis. Sick sinus syndrome manifested as marked sinus bradycardia (rate 28/min). As a result of sinus default, the A-V junction escapes and dissociates at a rate of 32/min. Whenever the sinus P wave lands on or beyond the T wave of the junctional beat, A-V conduction results (**ventricular capture**) with **RBBB aberration** in the top and bottom strips, without aberration in the middle strip.

Special Point. Of course it is impossible to distinguish marked sinus bradycardia from sinus exit block. For example, this manifest sinus rate of 28 min could be due to a sinus discharge rate of 56/min with 2 : 1 exit block.

267

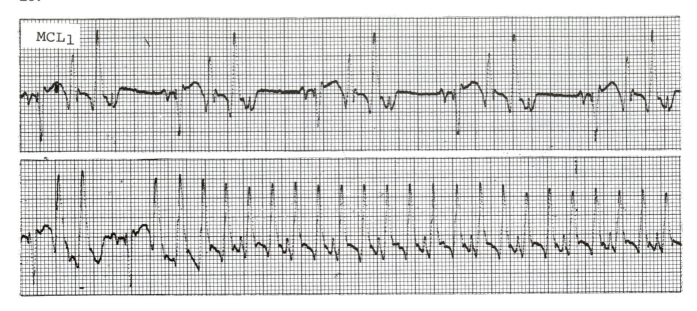

267

Diagnosis. **Top strip: sinus rhythm with paired left VPBs; retrograde conduction** to the atria follows the second of each pair (arrows). Bottom strip: the pair of extrasystoles is not followed by retrograde conduction, and after one more sinus beat, **left ventricular tachycardia** begins. Retrograde conduction follows the fourth beat of the tachycardia, and from then on there is 2 : 1 retrograde conduction (arrows).

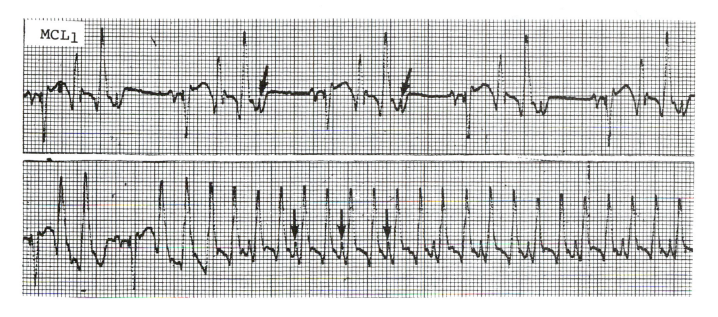

268

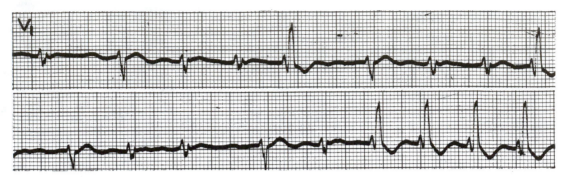

268

Diagnosis. **Atrial fibrillation; junctional tachycardia** (rate 125/min); 5:4 and 4:3 **Wenckebach** periods below junctional pacemaker; **rate-dependent RBBB.**

Special Points. At first the ventricular irregularity might be attributed to the atrial fibrillation. However, on more careful inspection, groups of three and four beats separated by the longest cycles become obvious, and within the groups there is progressive shortening of the ventricular cycles. These are clearly footprints of the Wenckebach phenomenon, and because the atria are fibrillating, the A-V Wenckebach must be occurring below a junctional pacemaker (see laddergram).

The degree of RBBB progressively increases as the cycle shortens in each group of beats; shrinkage of the S wave is often the earliest indication of developing RBBB.

The cycles of the last few beats in the bottom strip do not show progressive shortening, as one would expect with classic Wenckebach conduction. During Wenckebach-type conduction, it is not uncommon for the conduction interval to remain fairly constant for several beats (e.g., in Figure 118), and presumably that is what happens during these last few beats.

A fifth probable diagnosis is that there is some degree of A-V block above the junctional pacemaker, protecting it from disturbance by the fibrillatory impulses.

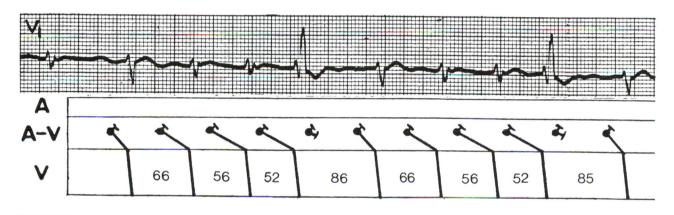

269

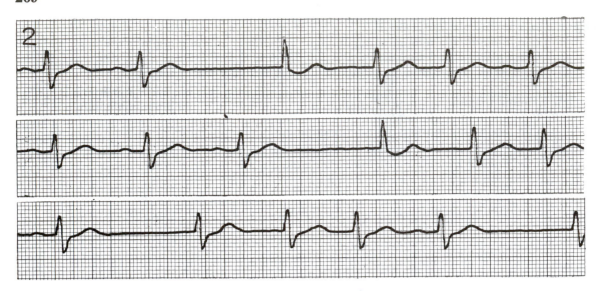

269

Diagnosis. **Sinus rhythm with Type II second-degree sinoatrial block** and potential second-degree Type I A-V block; **bundle-branch block.** The escape beats in the first and second strips that end the long cycles resulting from the sinoatrial block are presumably **junctional escape beats** in which intraventricular conduction has improved because of the longer diastolic rest. In the bottom strip, where the escape beats end slightly shorter cycles, the BBB is preserved in the escape beats.

Special Points. This is an elegant illustration of the reciprocal relationship between the R-P and the P-R intervals in A-V nodal block. Because this R-P/P-R reciprocity is demonstrable, the diagnosis of potential Type I second-degree A-V block is justifiable.

Because the shorter P-P intervals, as best one can measure them (arrows), appear to be similar and the long P-P intervals appear to be approximately twice the shorter intervals, by analogy with the cycle sequences in second-degree A-V block, the diagnosis of Type II sinoatrial block is warranted.

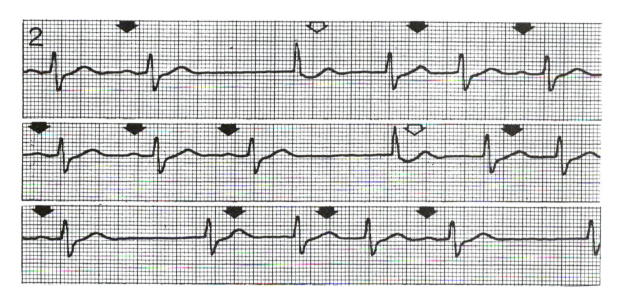

270

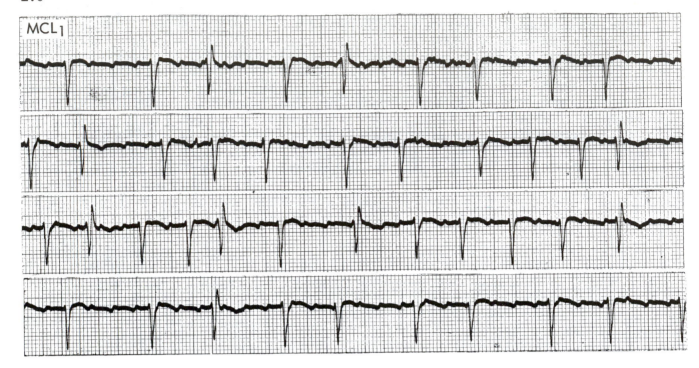

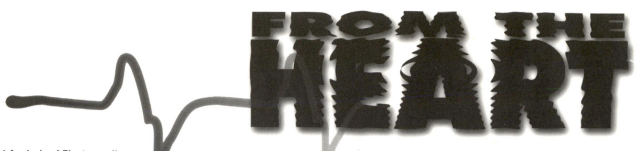

FROM THE HEART

Rapid Analysis of Electrocardiograms: A Self-Study Program
Second Edition

Emanuel Stein, MD, MPH, FACP, FACC, FCCP

A simple, straightforward writing style and ample illustrations augment this useful book, designed to provide the reader with a foundation in electrocardiography. Dr. Stein emphasizes a thoughtful, step-by-step approach with opportunities for self-assessment.

1992/414 pages/495 illustrations/1441-8/$24.95

Rapid Analysis of Arrhythmias: A Self-Study Program
Second Edition

Emanuel Stein, MD, MPH, FACP, FACC, FCCP

Get a step-by-step approach to recognizing both common arrhythmias and abnormal heart rhythms. Chapters include practice cardiac rhythms that challenge you to identify unlabeled arrhythmias, followed by the correct analysis and a clear explanation.

1992/230 pages/220 illustrations/1499-X/$26.95

Marriott's Practical Electrocardiography
Ninth Edition

Galen S. Wagner, MD

This classic for reading and interpreting ECGs is distinguished by an easily accessible style, outstanding coverage of ventricular aberrations and AV block, plus test tracings at the end of each chapter. "This is a high-quality book written with considerable clarity." — NEJM

1994/416 pages/291 illustrations/8604-9/$35.00

Pearls & Pitfalls in Electrocardiography: Pithy, Practical Pointers

Henry J.L. Marriott, MD, FACP, FACC

This unique book provides you with "tricks of the trade" to remember and pitfalls to avoid in electrocardiography. It covers all aspects of electrocardiography — arrhythmias, blocks and 12-lead tracings. **Pearls & Pitfalls** is a treasury of diagnostic gems and practical short cuts.

1990/158 pages/70 illustrations/1334-9/$30.00

Rhythm Quizlets: Self Assessment
Second Edition

Henry J.L. Marriott, MD, FACP, FACC

This new edition offers a convenient way to recognize arrhythmias in electrocardiograms and sharpen diagnostic skills. "Special Points" clarify pitfalls, and pertinent notes provide guidelines for therapy.

November 1995/about 800 pages/350 illustrations/5582-8/$32.95

Principles of Exercise Testing and Interpretation
Second Edition

Karlman Wasserman, PhD, MD; James E. Hansen, MD; Darryl Y. Sue, MD; Brian J. Whipp, PhD, DSc; and Richard Casaburi, MD, PhD

Including the most extensive discussion of mechanisms of exercise pathophysiology of any book in the field, this text follows a logical development from basic physiology through pathophysiology to practical application.

1994/489 pages/96 illustrations/1634-8/$62.00

CALL TOLL-FREE 1-800-638-0672 or return the attached reply card to: Williams & Wilkins, PO Box 1496, Baltimore, MD 21298-9724

Please send me:

_____ Marriott Pearls & Pitfalls in Electrocardiography (1334-9) $30.00

_____ Marriott Rhythm Quizlets, 2nd ed. (5582-8) $32.95

_____ Stein Rapid Analysis of Electrocardiograms (1441-8) $24.95

_____ Stein Rapid Analysis of Arrhythmias, 2nd ed. (1499-X) $26.95

_____ Wagner Marriott's Practical Electrocardiography, 9th ed. (8604-9) $35.00

_____ Wasserman et al Principles of Exercise Testing and Interpretation, 2nd ed. (1634-8) $62.00

Preview these texts for a full month. If you're not completely satisfied, return them at no further obligation (US only).

Williams & Wilkins
A WAVERLY COMPANY

INTERNET
E-mail: custserv@wwilkins.com
Home page: http://www.wwilkins.com/

Printed in US   9 95
MARRBI   I5B287   A

Payment options:

☐ Check enclosed (Plus $4.00 handling)
☐ Bill me (plus postage and handling)
☐ Charge my credit card (plus postage and handling)

_____ MasterCard   _____ VISA   _____ Am Express

_____
card #   exp. date

_____
signature/p.o. #

_____
name

_____
address

_____
city/state/zip

_____
phone #

_____
specialty/occupation

_____
fax #

CA, IL, MA, MD, ME, NY, and PA residents please add state sales tax. Prices subject to change without notice.

To order CALL Toll Free: 1-800-638-0672 Refer to #I5B287 when you order. FAX: 1-800-447-8438

270

Diagnosis. **Atrial flutter** (rate 255/min) with varying A-V conduction; **junctional parasystole** with **incomplete RBBB aberration.**

Special Points. The rSR″ pattern of the parasystolic beats suggests that they arise from an eccentric focus situated on the left side of the His bundle so that they are conducted more rapidly down that side than the right side (see diagram for Figure 150).

Note the 2 : 1 "filtering" at a higher level in the A-V junction, with Wenckebach periods develop-ing at a lower level (see laddergram); this is the usual mechanism in atrial flutter with varying ratios of A-V conduction.

Treatment. The average ventricular rate is about 92/min, and so there are two therapeutic options: slow the ventricular rate with digitalis, propranolol, or verapamil and hope that the resulting better perfusion will correct the arrhythmia or convert the atrial flutter by countershock. The parasystole by itself requires no therapy.

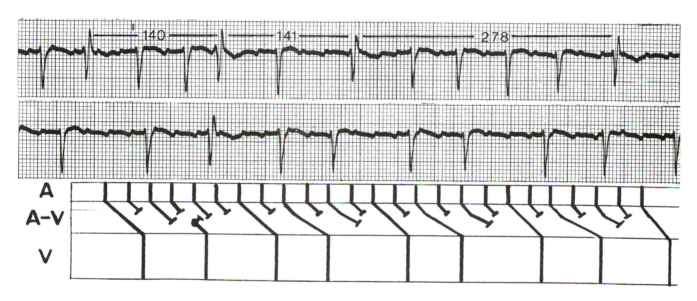

271

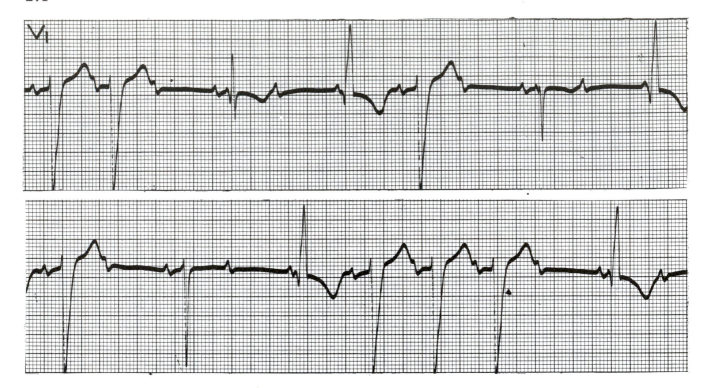

271

Diagnosis. **LBBB** with **Type II A-V block;
idioventricular escape rhythm** from the left
ventricle with frequent **fusion beats** (see figure).

Key: V = left ventricular idioventricular beats;
F = fusion between sinus and idioventricular impulses.

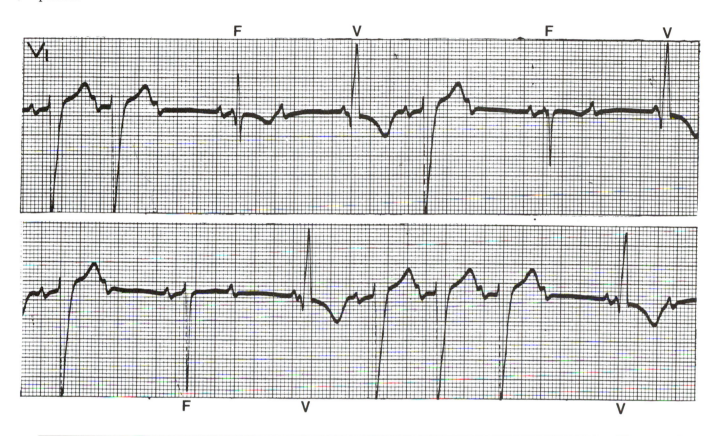

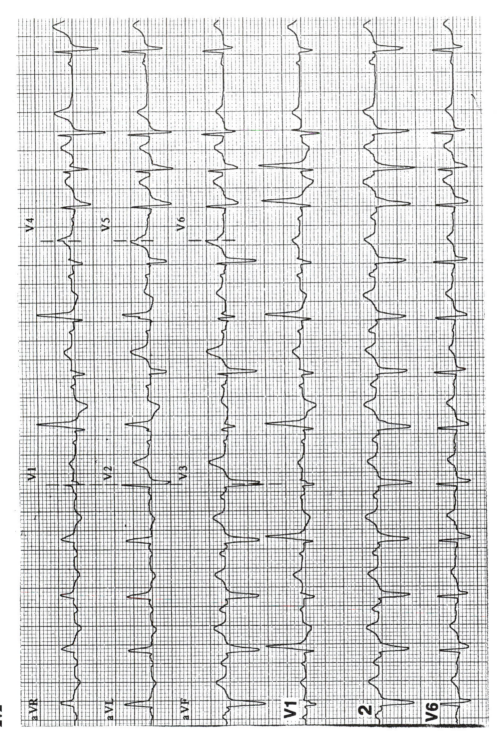

272

Diagnosis. **Sinus tachycardia** with **left anterior hemiblock** and alternating degrees of **RBBB**.

Special Point. Toward the end of the strip, the cluster of three beats demonstrates the importance of the preceding cycle in determining aberration (see Figure 212); beat 1 is aberrant be-cause of the prevailing 2 : 1 RBBB; beat 2 is aberrant because it ends a shorter cycle; beat 3, although it ends an identical short cycle, is not aberrant because it is preceded by a short cycle, that is, the cycle sequence 60 : 36 produces aberrancy but 36 : 36 does not.

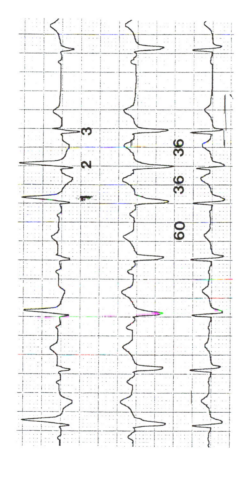

273

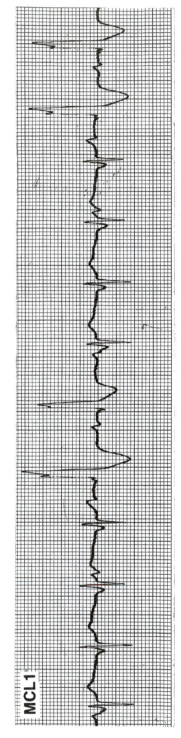

MCL1

274

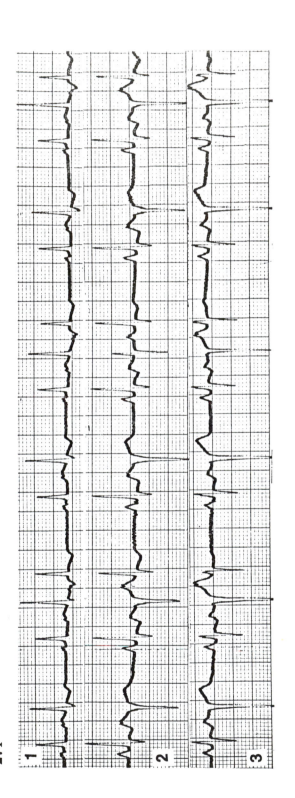

1

2

3

273

Diagnosis. Accelerated idioventricular rhythm (rate 90/min) dissociated from a sinus rhythm (rate 75/min) with paired **ventricular captures** showing prolonged PR intervals and **RBBB.** The second of each pair, with its q wave and less deep T wave, is a **fusion beat.**

274

Diagnosis. Sinus rhythm, with P waves suggesting P-pulmonale; single and paired **APBs,** the single ones and the first of each pair manifesting **left anterior hemiblock aberration.**

Special Point. Again this tracing eloquently illustrates the importance of the preceding cycle in determining aberration: each time there is a pair of APBs, the second of the pair shows no significant aberration, although it ends a cycle shorter than the preceding aberrant beat (compare with Figure 272).

275

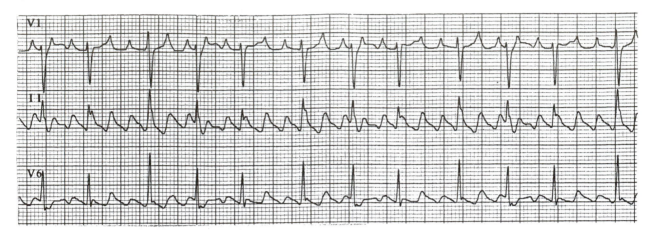

276

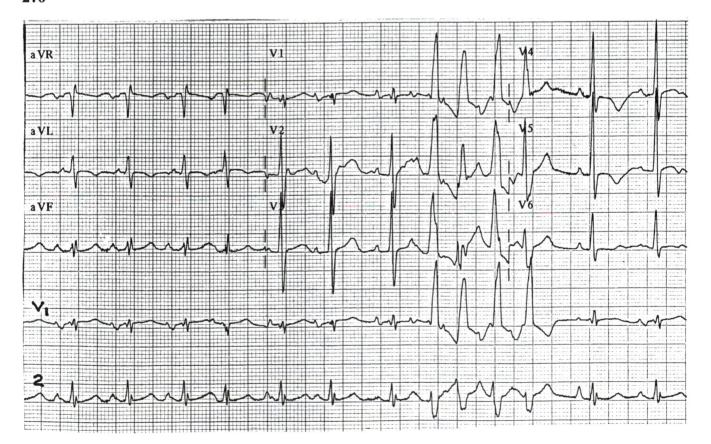

275

Diagnosis. Atrial flutter with varying A-V conduction (see laddergram).

Special Point. Whenever atrial flutter is associated with changing A-V conduction ratios, there is usually interplay between two levels of conduction. In this case there is 2 : 1 physiolgical "filtering" at an upper level, with 4 : 3 Wenckebach conduction at a lower level. Compare with Figures 126, 233, and 270.

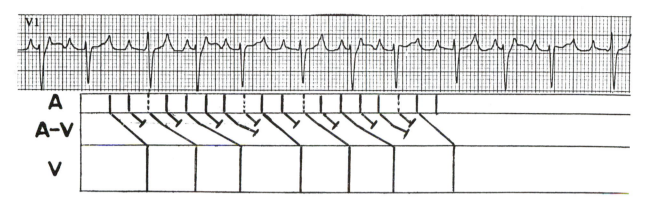

276

Diagnosis. The sinus rhythm is interrupted first by a single **APB** and then by a run of four APBs (i.e., atrial tacycardia) with atypical **RBBB aberration**.

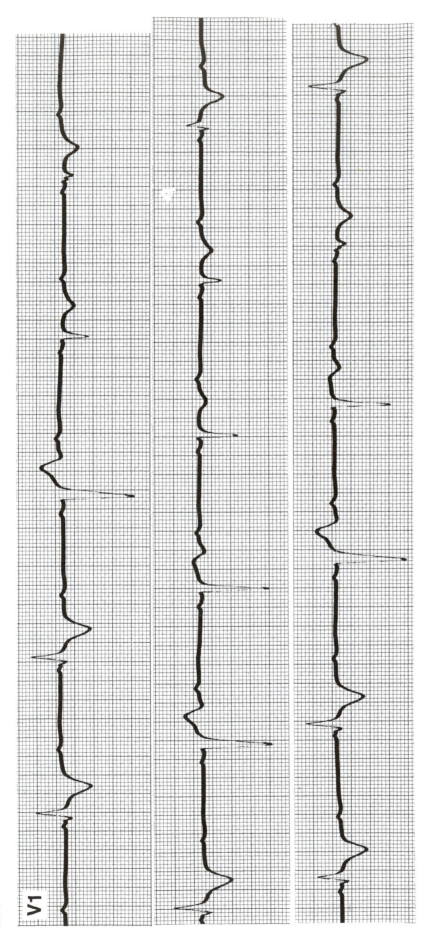

277

V1

277

Diagnosis. Sinus rhythm (rate 70/min) with **2 : 1**, probably Type II, **A-V block** and **LBBB**; a competing **idioventricular rhythm** from the left ventricle (e.g., first two beats in top and bottom strips) produces numerous **fusion beats.**

Special Point. When an ectopic ventricular pacemaker produces fusion beats with the sinus impulses in the presence of BBB on the same side as the ectopic center (here it is a left ventricular pacemaker in the presence of left BBB), the fusion QRSs may look remarkably normal (e.g., fourth beat in each strip).

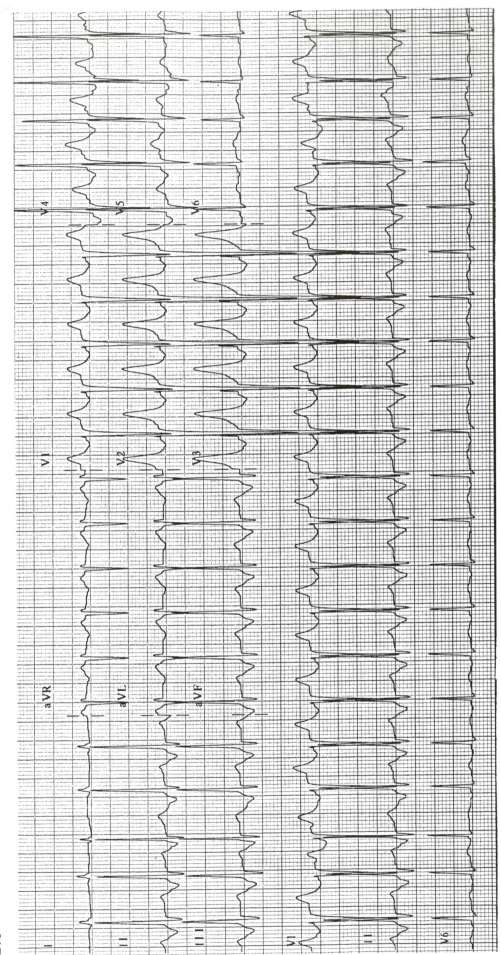

278

Diagnosis. **Reentrant supraventricular tachycardia** (rate 128/min) with R-P longer than P-R.

Special Point. The R-P longer than P-R makes a diagnosis of either the uncommon (fast to slow) form of A-V nodal reentrant tachycardia or orthodromic tachycardia using a slowly conducting retrograde accessory pathway.

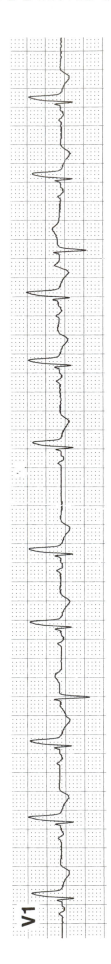

279 **V1**

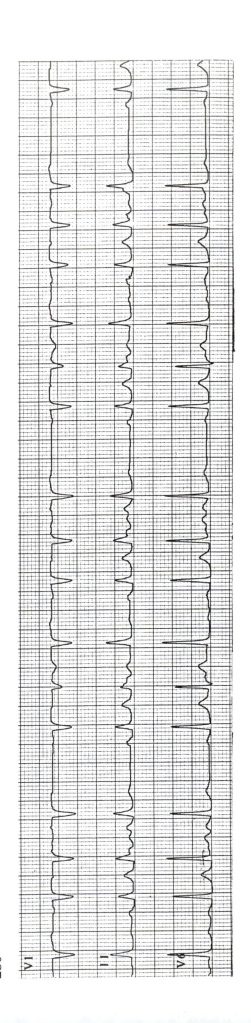

280

279   **Diagnosis.** Sinus rhythm with **RBBB** interrupted by two **APBs supernormally conducted** through RBB.

280   **Diagnosis.** Sinus rhythm with pairs and trios of **APBs**; when trios occur, the third APB is not conducted (see laddergram). (A trio of APBs constitutes the shortest definable paroxysm of atrial tachycardia).

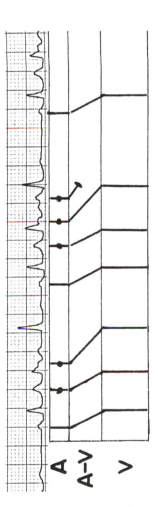

A

A–V

V

281

V₁

II

V₆

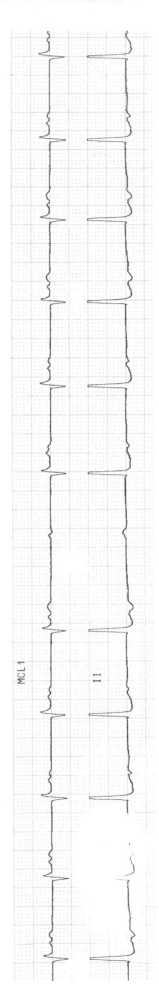

282

MCL 1

II

281

Diagnosis. **Atrial fibrillation** with a ventricular response rate of about 100/min; **rate-dependent RBBB.**

Special Point. That the RBBB is rate dependent is indicated by the improved conduction of beat 7, which ends one of the two longest cycles. Notice, however, that the bundle branch's response to rate is not consistent. This is not unusual in atrial fibrillation because the pattern of penetration into the A-V junction and the bundle branches is erratic and unpredictable. The much improved conduction manifested in beat 11 may be due to supernormal conduction through the RBB.

282

Diagnosis. **Potential Type I A-V block,** with markedly prolonged PR intervals (0.70 sec).

Special Point. Although this tracing is typical of A-V nodal block complete with "dropped" beat, there is no true Wenckebach phenomenon because there is no measurable increase in successive PR intervals and the atrial impulse that is not conducted to the ventricles is "dropped" because the P wave is slightly early (i.e., the P-P interval has shortened, and therefore the associated R-P has shortened to the point of failed A-V conduction).

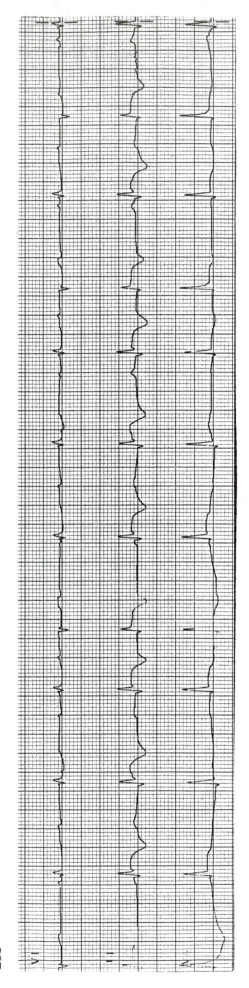

283

V1

II

V6

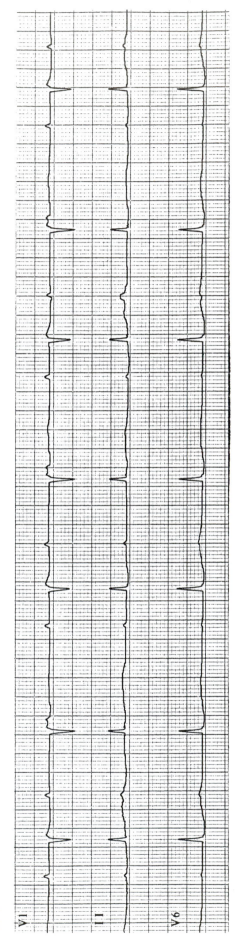

284

V1

II

V6

283

Diagnosis. Sinus tachycardia with **Type I A-V block** (in patient with acute inferior infarction) producing **A-V dissociation** with an **accelerated idionodal rhythm** (rate 62/min); 5th, 9th and 11th beats are ventricular captures.

Special Point. Note that the capture beats not only end shorter cycles but also have slightly changed QRSs.

284

Diagnosis. Sinus rhythm with **Type I A-V block** producing **3 : 2 Weckenbach periods** (see ladergram); **ventriculophasic sinus arrhythmia.**

Special Point. When, in the presence of A-V block, the sinus irregularity is such that the P-P intervals embracing a QRS are shorter than the P-P intervals that do not contain one, the sinus arrhythmia is said to be "ventriculophasic."

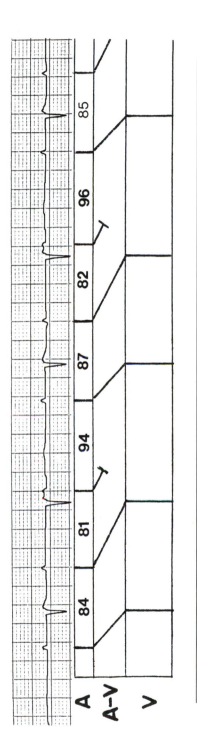

A
A–V
V

84 81 94 87 82 96 85

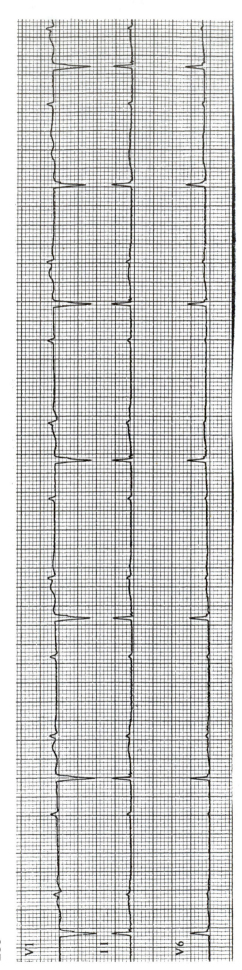

285

V1

II

V6

285

Diagnosis. **A 2 : 1 Type I A-V block** with **3 : 2 Wenckebach** toward end of strip (see ladergram).

Special Point. Note that the second P-R of the 3 : 2 Wenckebach reaches 0.80 sec.

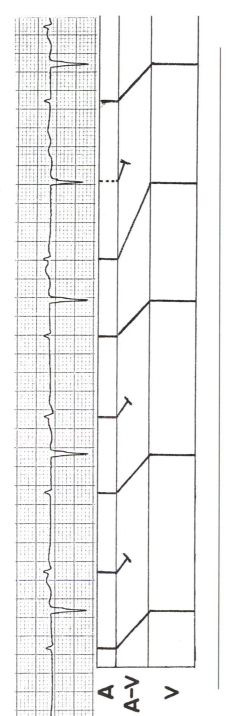

A

A–V

V

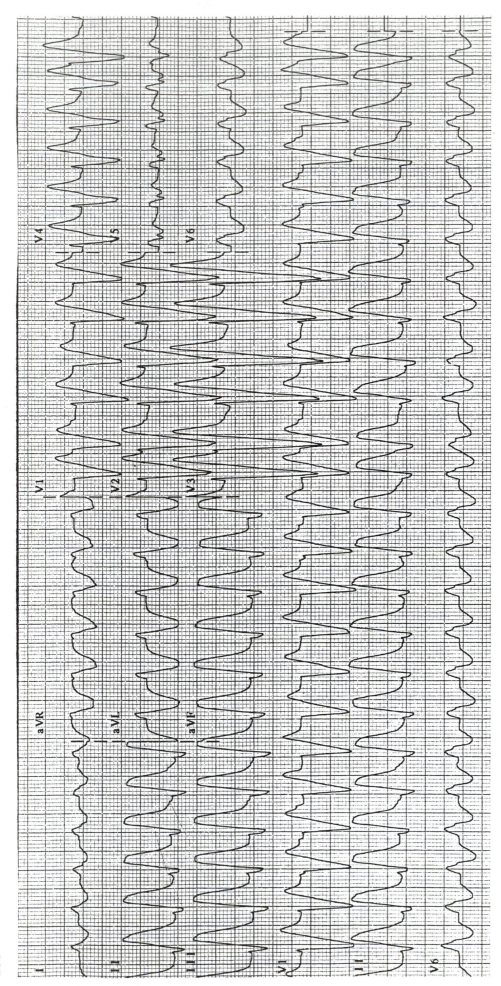

286

Diagnosis. Atrial tachycardia (rate 144/min) with **LBBB aberration** complicating an acute inferior infarction; **APBs.**

Special Point. The differential diagnosis here is clearly between ventricular tachycardia and supraventricular with left bundle-branch block. Because there is an acute infarction, one

naturally leans toward ventricular tachycardia, but the only morphological clue that is present, the slick downstroke to early nadir in V_1, favors LBBB. Diagnosis, however, is clinched by the demonstration of an unquestionable A-V Wenckebach (see laddergram).

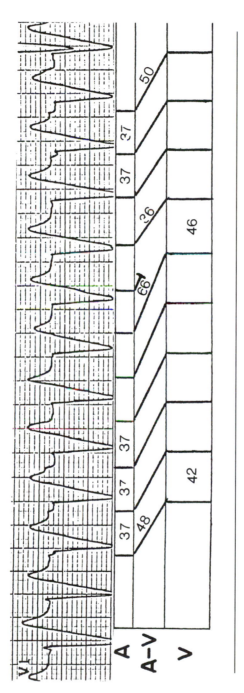

Index